DRUG REPAIR THAT WORKS

After eight years in the field of youth work and drug and alcohol counselling, Jost Sauer completed a Bachelor of Health Science (Acupuncture). He has been working as an acupuncturist since 1991 and lectured in traditional Chinese medicine for a decade at the Australian College of Natural Medicine in Brisbane. Jost also holds a Diploma in Oriental Massage (Tui-Na), certificates in Structural Balancing and Sports Injury Management, and undertakes ongoing studies in Body–Mind therapies. His interest in spirituality led to decades of research and training in spiritual healing under a master. Jost believes in 'silent teaching' and has spent over twenty years building his chi and spiritual awareness via a daily three-hour practice. He has conducted public seminars on traditional Chinese medicine, run meditation and chi workshops since 1992 and he is a regular contributor to health journals. Currently working as a therapist, Jost draws upon his acupuncture expertise, his years of intensive spiritual training and a life lived in harmony with the chi cycle. His treatments incorporate esoteric acupuncture to allow access to heightened levels of being.

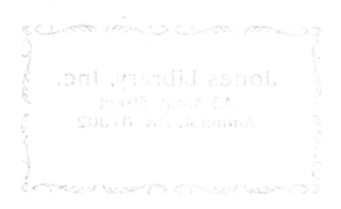

DRUG
REPAIR
THAT
WORKS

How to reclaim your health, happiness and highs

JOST SAUER

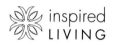

inspired
LIVING

ALLEN&UNWIN

First published in 2009

Inspired Living, an imprint of
Allen & Unwin
83 Alexander Street
Crows Nest NSW 2065
Australia
Phone: (61 2) 8425 0100
Fax: (61 2) 9906 2218
Email: info@allenandunwin.com
Web: www.allenandunwin.com

National Library of Australia
Cataloguing-in-Publication entry:

Sauer, Jost.

Drug repair that works : how to reclaim your health, happiness and highs / Jost Sauer.

978 1 74175 178 9 (pbk.)

Drug addiction--Treatment. Drug abuse. Drug withdrawal symptoms.

616.8606

Text Design by Lisa White
Set in 11.5/16pt Minion by Midland Typesetters, Australia
Printed and bound in Australia by Griffin Press

10 9 8 7 6 5 4 3

The paper this book is printed on is certified by the Programme for the Endorsement of Forest Certification scheme. Griffin Press holds PEFC chain of custody SGS - PEFC/COC-0594. PEFC promotes environmentally responsible, socially beneficial and economically viable management of the world's forests.

DEDICATION

Dedicated to Joachim Wagner (died 06/07/90), my best friend who introduced me to the magic realms, and to Sri Bhai Sahib Kirpal Singh Ji Gill who showed me the real magic and a path to never-ending highs.

NOTE ON TRADITIONAL CHINESE MEDICINE

In traditional Chinese medicine (TCM) the word 'organs' refers to an organ system, not the anatomical organ as understood in western medicine. The convention is to capitalise when referring to an organ in the Chinese context. For ease of reading, we are not applying this convention, nor the convention of discussing pairs of organs in the singular.

DISCLAIMER

CONTENTS

INTRODUCTION

Like it or not we are in the middle of a drug epidemic. What most people don't understand is that the 'drug problem' isn't confined to youth or the homeless. I see everything from amphetamine-addicted suburban mums and dope-dealing grannies, to pill-popping kids, many of whom think drugs are a natural part of life. Often medicated since primary school for attention deficit disorder or depression, and brought up on junk food, these teenage clients have already been living the life of a junkie for years. Drugs are also a daily reality for countless corporate employees, from lawyers to business executives. These high-achievers with fast cars and sharp suits are speed, cocaine and sometimes heroin users. Drugs make them feel powerful, fearless and able to work tirelessly for hours on end. They 'manage' their habit by exercising, eating well and maintaining a tan, but eventually the side-effects become unmanageable. Other clients are old hippies, still seeking spirituality and psychedelic experiences through drugs. I also see endless clients addicted to prescription medications: sleeping pills, antidepressants and the like.

It has been estimated that $400 billion a year is spent worldwide on recreational drugs, which represents eight percent of all international trade, about the same as tourism and the oil industry.[1] The common belief that youth or lower socioeconomic groups are the drug market cannot be true, because they simply don't have enough money. New research indicates that the fastest growing population of drug users in the US are white and middle-aged.[2] It seems the majority of drug users now are decent, respectable people who, despite their choice of intoxicants, earn a living and meet their responsibilities.

The illicit drug business is booming. The US is in the grip of a massive speed (methamphetamine) epidemic. Russia recently reported millions of drug addicts, and a new wave of cocaine abuse is spreading through Europe. In a recent book on heroin use in Britain, the author noted that in the city he worked in, heroin addicition had become such a mass phenomenon that the local city council was forced to send letters to each household asking them not to put used needles in their garbage bags.[3] There has even been a major revival in the use of magic mushrooms.[4] An American survey revealed an eleven percent increase in the use of ecstasy amongst school students.[5] Hundreds of millions of people consume cannabis and its use is increasing at a rate faster than that of other drugs.[6] A new amphetamine epidemic is currently sweeping Southeast Asia, with an estimated 18 million people using the drug.[7] As the young, increasingly westernised populations of China and India get on board the recreational drug wagon, the outcome will be globally devastating.

My many years as a therapist working with those struggling with drug dependency, as well as my own extensive drug experiences, have made me aware of the limitations of our current approach to drug issues, the inadequacy of many of our rehabilitation methods, and why, with the best intentions in the world, so many people continue to 'fall off the wagon'. The simple truth is that drugs can make you feel a whole lot better than you normally feel in everyday life—they can give you confidence, inspiration, a tangible sense of freedom and power, love and excitement. To assist those struggling with drugs, these aspects need to be acknowledged. Telling someone who has just had the most orgasmic experience possible that drugs are no good is laughable, because they know otherwise. Talk to any teenager who is using, and see what they have to say about current drug campaigns.

Alongside the euphoria that comes with drug use, there is also fear, frustration, anger, paranoia and violence. No matter how special the early drug experiences are, they can never be sustained. Over time it takes higher and higher doses of a drug to achieve less and less. Users find themselves in limbo—some part of them knows they're never going to reclaim their early highs, but at the same time the thought of going back to the mundane world is unbearable.

We have to present new and more effective programs and show people they can regain their health and passion for living, achieve their dreams, and continue to experience the highs after drugs. To do this, they need an integrated program that deals with their mental, physical and emotional needs, as well as those of their spirit, because drugs allow people to glimpse what the human spirit is capable of. This is the basis of the program I offer readers, alongside a collection of experiences, both personal and those of clients, to give them a detailed sense of the journey ahead.

My approach is informed by the astoundingly accurate insights traditional Chinese medicine offers those suffering mental, physical, emotional and spiritual depletion due to drug use. When I work with my clients we begin by building up the massively depleted organs, the source of much of the anger, confusion and even violence experienced by long-term users. As drugs use our life force (chi) to fuel each drug high, we also work on their daily routine, a straightforward diet that is nourishing and satisfying, bringing structure to their days, and also exercise to get their life force building again.

Many of those wanting to break their habit are consumed with guilt and shame, and too often families, friends and rehab clinics feed a person's sense of worthlessness. Regrettable experiences do happen on drugs, and users don't need others to tell them this. Too often the guilt and shame are so encompassing they fail to focus on the many valuable insights about themselves, their ideal relationships, their passions and the world that they may have gained on their journey. It is these insights that can help catapult people forward, because the best post-drug lives are about creating new ways of living and seeing, not about recreating an unsatisfactory past. You can use alcohol or drugs and live without being true to yourself, but once you give them up you can't.

When we dare to look deeper, whole new approaches become apparent. That is why I have devoted an entire section of this book to drug psychosis, for example. There is so much about psychosis we don't understand: we simply medicate it. However, treating the effects of drug abuse with other drugs is a short-term solution. Psychosis is much more logical than it seems. In traditional Chinese medicine, which developed over thousands of years of observation, there are very clear physical reasons why drug users hear voices or experience hallucinations. When a person's organ imbalances are corrected, the psychosis goes. An examination of their psychosis can also provide clues to the person's life mission.

It is these and other successful approaches I offer readers, so they can heal and create a new life. Written for users and their families, and for those working in drug recovery, *Drug Repair that Works* is a practical guide that deals with the complete picture, from where anger and confusion come from and why raw foods drain depleted bodies, to how to experience ongoing highs without drugs.

PART I:
A NEW APPROACH TO DRUGS

1 DISCOVERING DRUGS

My love affair with mood- and mind-altering substances began at fourteen. I would regularly take handfuls of my parent's tranquillisers and blissfully drift between worlds. At sixteen I discovered hashish and truly altered states. It launched me on the ride of a lifetime. LSD, magic mushrooms, mescaline, cocaine, heroin and amphetamines whipped me to the outer reaches of the universe or drew me into the depths of my soul. I thought the adventure would never end but it did, and badly. Speed addiction led to alcoholism and finally suicidal depression. Convinced that I'd done something wrong and wracked with guilt, I began working with drug-addicted youth in the social services. I thought helping others would make me feel better about myself, but eight years later I still felt just as bad.

Something needed to change. I went off to college to study traditional Chinese medicine, I became an acupuncturist and emerged with a shiny new version of myself. Determined no one was ever to find out about my drug past, I presented myself as a caring professional treating 'normal' disorders. When I opened my clinic everything went according to plan. Many of my patients were recreational drug users, but they came to me for acupuncture not drug issues, so I didn't have to go back into that anarchic territory. Then one day my past walked in the door and my life changed.

REDISCOVERING DRUGS

Jules was in his early twenties, very thin with heavily tattooed arms and legs, and a sore shoulder. I could tell he was a heavy drug user. He had a hunched body, too-pale skin, darkened teeth and the active but absent eyes of a speed user. Emotionally, he was highly wired and negative. Everything that was wrong in his life was someone else's fault. The speed was destroying his emotional outlook, health and spirit.

Despite my resolve to hide my past and my previous failures in helping drug addicts, I felt an overwhelming urge to do something about this so I launched into the session by talking openly of my experience with speed. I told him how much I had used, what side-effects it had and what caused them according to traditional Chinese medicine. Jules was stunned by my approach—as I was— but once he understood my past was far worse than his, he also saw that I couldn't be shocked, and the truth about his shoulder came out. He had been on a three-day binge that ended with a police chase and Jules falling off a high fence. Like the street kids I had worked with years ago, every second word was a four-letter one.

Jules was a classic example of everything I had run away from, but the strange thing was, I really enjoyed our interaction. I had never imagined this could happen. When I left youth work, I was totally disillusioned with the recovery scene. The people working in the system knew nothing about drugs or what it felt like to be without them when you were dependent. On my last project with addicted youth, the funding body expected my clients to be off drugs and back to normal within a certain period of time, but some of them had been addicts for years: they had never had a job, or even a glimpse of what society would call a normal life. They didn't want to stop drugs. Our programs were not working and no one knew why. There were no alternative programs to offer my clients either.

I had my own issues to deal with as well. Although I tried to look professional, underneath I suspected the real me was still a hopeless addict incapable of rational thought or action.

All that speed, as methamphetamine is usually referred to, had shaken my confidence in my own mental processes. For years my mind had felt like a box of firecrackers which could go off at a moment's notice. Random thoughts and ideas would explode within me, leaving a burned-out shell and drifting ashes. As one firecracker can set all the others off, if I was with another crazy drug user I could easily become that way as well.

This frequently happened when I was with the street kids. I'd fall back into the drug mind-set and involuntarily behave like one of them, laughing and carrying on about drugs in an inappropriate manner. They loved it but it didn't help them and I couldn't get my professional distance back. But now here I was sitting opposite Jules, a lit firecracker, and there was no sign of the fear, confusion and weakness that would usually have hit me by now in this therapeutic situation.

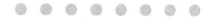

NEW APPROACHES

It took me a moment to register that this major shift was due to my discovery of traditional Chinese medicine. When I was in youth work it was all about psychology. We were supposed to find out what went wrong to make our clients take drugs, and then talk them through solutions. They were supposed to counter their drug cravings with positive thoughts. If it was that easy, I could have saved myself years of cravings and depression just by thinking positively.

If your body, or more specifically your organs, are depleted and destroyed by drugs or any other factor, you won't be able to process mental concepts. You won't believe affirmations or positive thinking. So to make change you need to start by rebuilding your depleted body.

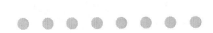

But traditional Chinese medicine had given me a new set of tools to work with that I knew would be effective for drug users. In traditional Chinese medicine, psychology and medicine are one. The focus is on the body, as it is through the body that we engage with physical reality. The body executes our dreams, desires and ideas.

If your body, or more specifically your organs, are depleted and destroyed by drugs or any other factor, you won't be able to process mental concepts. You won't believe affirmations or positive thinking. So to make change you need to start by rebuilding your depleted body.

Our organs are far more amazing than we imagine. While they have a range of physical functions, they also have spiritual and emotional functions. If the organs are operating at optimum level you will feel great physically, spiritually and emotionally. Jules was using speed because he wanted to feel good. Speed makes you feel very, very good, because it artificially enhances the ability of your organs to function. High on speed, you feel immortal, exhilarated and euphoric.

Each organ is connected with a different emotion. The lungs are connected with freedom and spontaneity. If they operate at peak level you can embrace change, let go of the past and see an exciting future. The heart generates feelings of love, inspiration and joy. The liver is connected with happiness and inner energy (chi) flow. A healthy spleen gives you a strong sense of boundaries and allows you to trust people and want to communicate with them. The kidneys provide willpower and fearlessness. If you put all this together it provides an insight into how a speed high feels. It is also an insight into how we should all feel without speed.

Unfortunately, constantly forcing the organs to work at this level with drugs is damaging, so in between the great highs you begin to feel terrible. By

ORGAN	POSITIVE EMOTIONAL ATTRIBUTES	NEGATIVE EMOTIONAL ATTRIBUTES
Lungs	Spontaneity, letting go, living in the now	Loss, grief, living in the past
Heart	Love, inspiration, joy	Shock, panic, depression
Liver	Happiness, energy flow, direction in life	Frustration, anger, inability to move, bitterness
Spleen	Boundaries, clarity of thought, trust, vitality	Confusion, scattered mind, fatigue
Kidneys	Willpower, fearlessness, vigour	Fear, weakness, helplessness

the time I quit drugs, my organs were no longer healthy and were not able to generate positive feelings. Due to depleted lungs I was overwhelmed with loss and grief. My heart made me feel depressed. My liver left me angry and frustrated. My spleen filled me with confusion and paranoia, and my kidneys made me feel fearful and weak. At this point you tend to take more drugs so all the bad feelings go away, but it just makes everything worse because you are depleting your organs even more. This was the emotional territory that Jules was heading into.

The healing of our organs allows resolution of emotional issues.

When you are feeling angry, bitter, frustrated, paranoid, empty and confused from drug use, you can talk to counsellors, psychologists or psychiatrists until the cows come home but unless you restore health to your organs, things will not change. I knew this from my own experience. I had been in a much worse state than Jules. He was still able to interact with people. Towards the end of my speed-taking days I couldn't talk to anyone, let alone look them in the eye. By committing to a lifestyle that would heal my organs, my emotions eventually became more positive. Gradually I found myself feeling more optimistic about life and wanting to interact with people. But I had no idea that I could achieve such emotional balance; that I would be able to speak about my drug use without turning into a psychological mess.

REIGNITING THE AFFAIR

I finished the session with Jules by giving him acupuncture to alleviate his shoulder pain. Then I wrote a program for him to develop strength and health. I suggested he have as many warm cooked meals as possible and a good amount of protein as drug users are usually protein deficient. Ideally he would add nutritional supplements as well. His exercise program included some stretching as soon as he woke, followed with endurance work and weights. I also directed him to a local tai-chi school to learn about his own inner energy (chi) flow. All of this would help him understand what the drugs were doing and how to continue the journey of discovery without drugs.

He left in an optimistic state and I did too. That night I actually went home excited and inspired. It was the first day I felt truly fulfilled since I had given up drugs. I felt alive again. Part of this was the realisation that my experiences with drugs, my recovery, and my intimate knowledge of traditional Chinese medicine could be used to help others.

The consultation with Jules reignited my unfinished affair with drugs. It made me see that I still had a passion for altered states. If I combined that with my passion for traditional Chinese medicine I could work with my two favourite things and help people. Over the next few months Jules' life improved dramatically. It was one of the most rewarding cases I had had since starting work as a therapist.

2 USING DRUGS

By building my organs and cultivating my inner energy (chi) my whole life changed. The gradual improvement in my lungs meant I could start to accept my past. This is important because otherwise you can get caught up in permanent regret and blame. As my heart became healthier, my depression was replaced with excitement and I felt inspired about life again. A healthier liver meant I was no longer frustrated, bitter and stuck. I now had strong direction in life, my energy flowed and I experienced happiness. Because of my improved spleen function, I had boundaries. I was clear about who I was and what my purpose in life was and I wanted to bond with people again. By healing my kidneys I had the willpower to set goals and conquer the fear of starting new projects. Healthy kidneys also provided me with a sense of having 'deep roots' in life.

COMING CLEAN

My improved organ function explained my sudden desire to engage with Jules and share what I knew about drugs, even though he reminded me of my painful past. Now that my organs were healthy, I could speak about the crazy escapades of my drug past but keep my feet firmly planted on the ground.

After Jules, I started to attract more clients with drug issues. The more open I was about my past, the more open they were and the more successful the outcomes. Then I began lecturing at a college of natural medicine, and wrote my first book *Higher and Higher* in which I admitted my drug past. In one fell swoop I went from keeping my past buried to making it public. It was the best thing I ever did. Making sure the decent folk never found out who I really was had been exhausting. Being able to be myself was such a relief.

In body–mind medicine, therapy is considered to be a two-way process. You attract what you are to deal with. I was getting a very strong message to use my drug past, because now all my patients wanted help with drug issues.

THE DRUG-USING DEMOGRAPHIC

Initially I treated a lot of young hard-drug users. They dabbled in crime and lived outside the rules of society. In a way I picked up where I had left off years before in youth work but, as I was now getting positive results, it resolved some of my past failure issues.

Ex-hippies who had become successful business people were the next group. Now approaching middle-age, they had become part of the establishment they once fought against. Many couldn't stop smoking marijuana because it was the only way they could keep in touch with past dreams and recapture the feelings of magic and mystery they'd once had. But marijuana wasn't delivering the goods anymore. Instead they were becoming increasingly frustrated and cynical about life. You can't rely on drugs to keep delivering the dream. Drugs are temporary and you need to find a permanent method of putting the magic back into life.

You can't rely on drugs to keep delivering the dream. Drugs are temporary and you need to find a permanent method of putting the magic back into life.

I also treated many of the 'ecstasy generation'—people in their twenties and early thirties. Environmentally conscious and compassionate, they longed for spiritual fulfilment and a psychedelic element in their lives. Ecstasy provided them with instant and powerful experiences of this. I also saw professional business people who used drugs, including speed and cocaine, as performance enhancers.

My clients were all using different drugs for different reasons, so a common aspect of my treatment was identifying what the drug delivered for each individual and working out other means of meeting this need. If you are going to take a drug away, you need to replace it with something that can fulfil its role or the person will return to the drug.

Another group of clients I see are teenage drug users, fifteen- or sixteen-year-olds who have often been taking drugs since they were ten or eleven. These are normal school children from normal families trying to give up drugs at the age I discovered drugs. When asked why they use drugs they generally shrug and say, 'Everybody does it.' When we talk about what they like about drugs, they refer to fantasy computer games or books. They want to be in that world. When parents, teachers or other adults tell them it is just a dream, they use marijuana, ecstasy or other drugs to try to make it reality.

> If you are going to take a drug away, you need to replace it with something that can fulfil its role or the person will return to the drug.

Most of these young clients have been to counsellors or doctors prior to seeing me. These professionals focused on where the child had gone wrong, but maybe our generation are the ones who 'went wrong'. We were supposed to have changed the world. In the 1960s and 70s hallucinogenic drugs showed us this was possible. We saw what a magical place the world could be. We felt brotherhood and love. We didn't follow up on what the drugs had shown us, though. We didn't make it real. Eventually our visions went but the drug-taking stayed. We contributed to an environment in which young people would turn to drugs to feed their souls.

GROUP MEMORY

According to biologist Rupert Sheldrake, if a lot of people start doing, thinking or practising something different, new patterns of behaviour can spread faster than would otherwise be possible. Laboratory experiments have shown that if rats of a particular breed learn a new trick in one location, rats of that breed are able to learn the same trick faster in other locations without any obvious communication between the groups.[1] Mainstream science cannot explain this phenomenon.

In Sheldrake's theory, each individual contributes to the collective memory of their species, and modifies the group memory or morphic field. The next generation born into that modified field then adopts the new behaviour without having to learn it.[2] These fields apply to all aspects of our lives, even intelligence. Sheldrake points out that our IQ has been steadily rising as each successive generation absorbs learning from past generations. I wonder whether the drug-taking that began in the 1960s formed a morphic field—or powerful group mind-set—that contributed to the subsequent boom in recreational drug use.

The rave phenomenon of the 1980s, fuelled by the drug ecstasy, is now considered the largest youth movement in Britain's history.[3] As with the hippies before them, many of its followers have continued using drugs. Now the next generation of drug users, the young teenagers, have appeared. Younger again and more numerous than the ravers, they view drug use as something 'everyone does'. They also say 'drugs make sense of everything'. My friends and I rejected the values and limitations of the material world when we took drugs, but we didn't do it to make sense of anything. This is a new development.

> While young people are born into an environment in which drug-taking is normal, they also seem to have inherited the expanded consciousness drugs introduced to previous generations.

If there is a morphic field for intelligence, perhaps there is also a morphic field for consciousness. While young people are born into an environment in which drug-taking is normal, they also seem to have inherited the expanded consciousness drugs introduced to previous generations. The world of magic, creativity, freedom and excitement that they expect to be living in was the world we all imagined and talked about back in the 1960s. Maybe drugs 'make sense of everything' for these kids because drugs allow them to feel they are living in that world. Perhaps if we had changed the world and set up societies based on love and equality, they wouldn't need drugs.

Then again, perhaps changing the world wasn't our responsibility. If people take drugs to feel magic, expansion, creativity and freedom, and if these states 'make sense', the solution to the drug problem is to change our inner worlds. If we had done this after we took drugs, we would have created a very different morphic field for the following generations. The good news is that it is not too late to do this. In traditional Chinese medicine it is said that we see the world through our organs. Our organs can deliver everything drugs can, even 'make the world different' and much, much more.

> Maybe drugs 'make sense of everything' for these kids because drugs allow them to feel they are living in a world of creativity freedom and excitement.

> If people take drugs to feel magic, expansion, creativity and freedom, and if these states 'make sense', the solution to the drug problem is to change our inner worlds.

3 A NEW APPROACH TO RECOVERY

Being immersed in the drug world again made me aware of how different current recreational drug use is from that of the 1960s counter-culture. The drugs are more powerful. Post-drug symptoms are manifesting much more quickly than in the past. I see clients now, like Jules, who within a year or so of hard drug use have the side-effects that it took me many years to develop.

Attitudes towards drug use have also changed significantly. The majority of clients I see have no interest in feeling guilty for taking drugs and don't relate to recovery programs based on that concept. Many come out of rehab and go straight back to drugs. They need a new non-judgemental recovery model expressed in a language that they can relate to. This model must address body, mind and spirit, because drugs affect us on all these levels.

I could never accept the idea that the effects of recreational drugs are due to alterations in brain chemistry. Scientists locate the mind in the brain, but there is no research which conclusively shows the higher levels of the mind—thoughts, feelings and rich subconscious elements—are located in brain tissue.[1] Explaining the blissful euphoria and bonding of ecstasy, the multidimensional tripping of LSD and the feelings of immortality you get from speed as alterations in brain chemistry does not make sense. When you are in those states you *feel* it in the body. In traditional Chinese medicine the emotions and higher levels of mind are housed in the body, in the organs. Each of the organs has a physical presence but also an immaterial presence. It has an invisible field around it. I believe most drug damage occurs on this non-material or astral body. A special form of acupuncture, combined with spiritual training, allows repairs to be made on this level of our being.

THE MAGIC OF TRADITIONAL CHINESE MEDICINE

Drugs create non-ordinary states of consciousness that are mystical or transcendental. Traditional Chinese medicine can acknowledge these states because it grew out of early Chinese alchemy, which aimed to understand the formation and workings of the cosmos.[2] Traditional Chinese medicine continued to develop over four thousand years. There was no separation of body and mind, and no rejection of spirit.

In traditional Chinese medicine, spirit plays as important a role as body or mind. There are acupuncture points that are specifically used to open a person to spiritual awareness.[3] All illness also has spiritual implications. The therapeutic tool is chi, our invisible life force. Chi is also the basic substance from which the cosmos is made. The ancient Chinese scholars described it as very minute particles in continuous motion. They also described it as the motive force in the transformation of things.[4] This means in traditional Chinese medicine *everything* can change, everything can be transformed.

There are 361 acupuncture points on our body and these are like doorways that direct life force or chi into our internal organs. The acupuncture points also link us to the external universe. In some schools of thought, there is a connection between acupuncture points and different planets, constellations and even the ley lines—the lines of energy—that cross the earth.[5] Practitioners of traditional Chinese medicine can draw the life force from heaven and earth and use it to help heal the patient. Traditional Chinese medicine is poetic, simple, complex and practical all at once.

RECAPTURING PSYCHEDELIC EXPERIENCES THROUGH BODYWORK

Traditional Chinese medicine is also subtle, and it aims at preventing sickness. The idea is to have treatment regularly to maintain health and improve longevity. But westerners wait until they are ill before seeking help, then they expect instant results. Pharmaceutical drugs deliver this, but with traditional Chinese medicine it may take longer.

Drug users are accustomed to instant highs and instant change, so as clients of mine they needed a profound experience of change in the first session. To achieve this I added bodywork, a technique of working with the body to go straight to the core of deep-seated blockages. Basically, it allows you to engage with the psychology of the person without the need for lengthy conversations. In bodywork you use your fingertips or knuckles to push along the limbs in the direction of the energy flow. It is a powerful technique and creates a real sense of change.

I combined this technique with acupuncture on the points that allow clients to enter a dream-like state while fully conscious. This frees deep-seated issues and allows them to come to the person's conscious mind. As the person is in an altered state and distanced from daily life, they can experience and process feelings in a state of total acceptance. Feelings that might be too painful or difficult to put into words could arise, be resolved and dissolve. The client can also have dream-like images and visions streaming through their mind. People often describe seeing themselves in other times and places in different bodies. Many would get off the massage table thinking they had had a drug flashback.

LETTING GO OF JUDGEMENT

Drug users are a unique kind of client. For them therapy isn't just about releasing stored pain, because daily life keeps adding more pain. They have to face constant negativity about their drug use from families, friends and the media. Everything you hear about drugs is negative. Even if you have given up drugs, it still feels as if every bad drug story is about you.

This was brought home to me recently when I watched a reality television program in which a cameraman followed addicts of the drug ice, an intense crystalline form of methamphetamine. They were in a desperate state. Their teeth were rotting and they were seriously delusional. They were filmed obsessively sorting through rubbish bins, living in squalor and picking at their open sores.

I could barely watch the show because it made me so uncomfortable—not because of the content, but because this type of programming holds drug users up to public condemnation. After seeing that show I had feelings of low self-esteem and hopelessness that I couldn't shake. I realised it had taken me right back to how I had felt as a drug user: a leper and an outcast. My reaction caught me by surprise. I hadn't used drugs for decades but, like most drug users who have been demonised, I must still have been carrying remnants of guilt and shame. It was hard to regain my equilibrium and sense of self-worth. I could only imagine how bad current drug users would have felt watching that footage. I believe this sort of media coverage drives drug users further into drug use and destruction. It feeds a negative cycle.

The majority of my clients are initially hesitant to speak openly about their drug use even when they know that I too was a heavy user. Most assumed that I would either be making them admit that they had done something wrong or that I would probe them to find out what had gone wrong to make them take drugs in the first place, as this was the way health practitioners had treated them in the past. This was also what had happened to me.

The countless therapists and counsellors I saw in order to try to understand my post-drug pain, emptiness and depression all had a judgemental approach without even realising it. Their work was based on the assumption that you

> Drug users are a unique kind of client. For them therapy isn't just about releasing stored pain, because daily life keeps adding more pain. They have to face constant negativity about their drug use from families, friends and the media.

have to have serious problems to take drugs. I listened to them because, like many ex-drug users, my organs were so weak that I sought structure, purpose and meaning in other people's ideas. Everything they said was based on theory, but drugs are all about *experience*. It never occurred to these professionals that I took drugs because I *loved* the way they made me feel. This should be the key issue in recreational drug recovery treatment programs.

Ancient Chinese Taoist philosophies say there is no such thing as good and evil. Things and people are simply what they are. I decided that the basis for my work would be that drugs are what they are, neither good nor bad (which of course is the truth) and that the people who take them are what they are as well. If drugs and drug users are neutral, there is no point having a war on them—it would be like declaring war on Switzerland.

FORBIDDEN FRUIT

There is a misconception that people take drugs because they are forbidden, and therefore more attractive. I don't agree. Drug users don't want drugs because they are forbidden, they want them because they make you feel good. They want the excitement, euphoria, action, confidence, laughter, stress relief and the many other positive states drugs provide. Drug users need a new therapeutic approach that changes the way they view themselves and their drug use. This is done by working with the transformative potential of their past drug experiences.

Drug users need a new therapeutic approach that changes the way they view themselves and their drug use. This is done by working with the transformative potential of their past drug experiences.

● ● ● ● ● ● ● ●

This way people can build positively on their past, rather than feeling guilty about it. I had always been fascinated by the ancient Chinese alchemists who sought to utilise the energies and properties of various substances to ascend to higher states of being beyond the limits of human freedom.[6] Recreational drugs are the most powerful substances on the planet, and hold tremendous transformative potential. When I tap into a client's past from this perspective, we can convert all their negativity and pain into something magical.

4 SPEED, CREATIVITY AND SELF-DEVELOPMENT

My first client to experience the new approach I was developing to drug recovery was Robyn, an attractive 24-year-old. She was well presented in a nicely tailored beige suit, white collared shirt and hair pulled back in a neat ponytail. She managed a hair salon.

Robyn started smoking marijuana at the age of fifteen and within two years was smoking it every day. At nineteen she discovered speed and before long was injecting it daily. After a few years of this, the side-effects got so bad she had to give up. Since then Robyn desperately craved speed but she saw what it had done to her friends—the aggressive behaviour, the trouble with police and the loss of direction in life—and didn't want that. But without speed she felt she couldn't cope with life.

TAKING THE PULSE

I began by taking her pulse the Chinese way which, as well as enabling you to diagnose the state of all the organs, gives symbolic information about what is going on in the client's life. As soon as I started, in my mind's eye I saw an image like an angry little daredevil in a box, suggesting unexpressed anger. I then searched the pulse for the organ related to that, and my attention was drawn to the spleen, which was clearly deficient. This meant Robyn would have no energy to express herself, and would be confused about boundaries.

As that image faded, my vision clouded. It was as if I was looking through muddy, swirling water. The 'dirty water' indicated Robyn had no clarity about her life or her spirit was not clear. I asked her if she had the sensation of a film between herself and reality, and she said yes. When I then saw a forest of huge trees around me, I knew her condition was also connected with the wood element and its associated organ, the liver. This was an indication that Robyn was frustrated at not living in accord with her true direction. Overall, the pulse revealed organ deficiencies that would be causing a lack of motivation, an inability to get up in the morning, anxiety, sleep disorders, shortness of breath and panic attacks. Robyn would have little patience and be highly irritable.

When I listed these symptoms Robyn was stunned at how accurate the diagnosis was. She was also relieved to learn these symptoms could all be corrected with ongoing acupuncture and professionally administered Chinese raw herbs. In traditional Chinese medicine, the study of herbs is a refined art. The herbs are very potent. They enter specific meridian systems and go straight to the targeted organ, building strength, restoring health and correcting symptoms rather than masking symptoms as pharmaceutical drugs do.

> Overall, my pulse diagnosis on Robyn revealed organ deficiencies that would be causing a lack of motivation, an inability to get up in the morning, anxiety, sleep disorders, shortness of breath and panic attacks. Robyn would have little patience and be highly irritable.

Robyn began talking about how bad things were and how her life was on a downward spiral. To get her onto the track of finding the positives in her past drug experiences, I needed to find what she had loved about drugs, and see how we could recapture that.

As Robyn had begun using drugs at fifteen, I asked what her dreams were when she was a teenager. She seemed a bit thrown by this and looked uneasy, then admitted that as a teenager she didn't feel like she fitted in. She hated school. She was bisexual and wanted to be expressive but had to suppress this desire. Her first taste of marijuana provided an instant connection to her true self. Now we were getting somewhere.

When I asked what she meant by 'connection', she said that along with drugs she discovered the psychedelic music and culture of the 1960s. Rock stars and folk singers became her role models, because they lived by their own rules with no inhibition. Robyn associated drugs with delivering that feeling of freedom, so she made drugs her lifestyle. She joined a psychedelic trance band, wore dreadlocked multicoloured hair and outrageous theatrical clothes. She styled people's hair at raves and festivals and felt as if she was living her dream. She pushed up a sleeve and showed me a beautiful Japanese-style full-arm tattoo.

She was now speaking passionately about herself and her life, and looked active and engaged. This was the real Robyn. I explained that drugs make your dreams seem tangible and concrete, but when you stop the drugs, you lose the connection to your dreams and your true self becomes inaccessible again. That was why she now woke up feeling empty and depressed. Robyn said that in the past she would have done a line of speed before getting out of bed, to counter the emptiness and motivate her to move.

WAKING UP FOR SPEED

I said, 'So you used to wake up for speed?' Robyn agreed, looking very embarrassed. I explained she had done that to experience herself as she would like to be and that speed had, in fact, been fulfilling the role of a daily spiritual practice for her. Robyn looked shocked. She said that she thought she had wasted years of her life and wished she hadn't done any drugs. When I asked her what she would have done if she hadn't taken drugs she couldn't answer. I had also assumed my years spent using drugs were wasted, but I couldn't say what I would have done instead. Maybe there was a reason.

Robyn was also concerned that she had wasted thousands of dollars on drugs. She had been shooting up approximately $100 of speed per day. That came to $73 000 over two years. Adding in the weekend extras of ecstasy and marijuana, the total was at least $100 000. I wrote it down on a piece of paper. Robyn sat staring at the figure. Before she could speak I suggested that rather than thinking of it as wasted money, she should view it as having paid for years of intense therapy. Like therapy, drugs provide us with a conscious experience of the subconscious mind. They reveal information about our true desires that is not usually accessible to us. These revelations are invaluable because they can help you define your purpose and destiny. Drugs do not bring out what is not there. Drugs show us what immense potential we have.

Robyn needed to make sure she got her money's worth from her years of drug-taking by making that knowledge work for her, not against her. The way to do this was to reprogram herself by understanding that on speed she had developed powerful reference points for life. Speed had shown her what she wanted to be and she had to commit to recapturing that. If she followed up on these insights she wouldn't have wasted her time or money.

> Like therapy, drugs provide us with a conscious experience of the subconscious mind. They reveal information about our true desires that is not usually accessible to us.

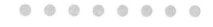

My next question was why she dressed the way she did. Robyn said she was worried about what the customers thought of her. She felt weak and depressed and did not want to attract attention to herself. She wanted to blend in. I had done this too after drugs. Initially speed is such a powerful drug that it forces all your organs to function at peak level. You feel fantastic, free, powerful and excited, and you want to express yourself in every way possible. On speed your organs give you such support you feel safe being different from everyone else.

In the early eighties, at the height of my speed days, I had a multicoloured mohawk haircut. I wore a lot of jewellery and make-up. My clothes were

> On speed your organs give you such support you feel safe being different from everyone else.

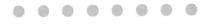

outlandish. It took me hours to get ready before I went out. Because my organs were operating at optimum level, I was liberated from social conditioning. This is how we should feel naturally without drugs. After giving up speed my organs were weak. I felt grief, loss, confusion, anxiety and fear. I didn't know who I was. I had nothing to express anymore. I was paranoid about what people thought of me and lived through the eyes of others. I cut my hair, took off my jewellery and wore bland clothes.

Robyn's appearance had been a form of expression for her, so it was important for her to reclaim this. She had to be creative in her clothes, jewellery and hair, and present herself to her clients as the eccentric free spirit she really was. To achieve this she needed to give her organs what they required so they could operate perfectly again, and so she could feel safe being herself. Instead of forcing this through drugs, she had to create it through a lifestyle of exercise, medicinal food, herbs and therapy.

I worked out a new daily practice to correct what she didn't like about herself and help her become the way she would like to be. Instead of struggling out of bed, drinking lots of coffee, chain-smoking cigarettes and snacking on high-sugar cereals on her way to work, Robyn would start each day with some yoga and kick-boxing. This would give her the skills to work with her inner energy flow and build feelings of wellbeing. Instead of nibbling on junk food in between clients, which further damages the spleen, she would stop for proper meal breaks and eat well to nuture the spleen. She would also follow up our consultation with regular acupuncture to counter her anxiety, sleep disorders and panic attacks.

I suggested that her new daily guiding principle be 'I know there is more to life than a nine-to-five existence, and I'm going to have that again. I will build my body, mind and spirit so I can live the way I want to in accord with how right it felt when I was on drugs. I will expand, I will discover, I will focus on recapturing the way I felt at the height of the great drug days. Drugs were only the first step on my journey, now I will chase the real highs'.

As I spoke the air around me was charged. I could feel the familiar spiritual presence and guidance with me when I did acupuncture, so I knew a healing energy was present. Robyn's eyes were changing. Her excitement and inspiration were rising. I knew she could feel what I did.

Robyn left determined to make changes in her life. She understood that speed had shown her what she could be by revealing the potential of her organs. Her goal was to recapture that without speed by building up her organs. Over time, as her organs became more healthy, she became more comfortable with being herself. She started speaking openly about her sexuality and her struggle with drugs. To her surprise this didn't meet with condemnation or judgement from others. On the contrary, people were supportive and more open about themselves.

After the session with Robyn I felt uplifted as well. This was the first time I had focused purely on counselling since my youth work days, and it had been far more effective than it was then. When I was a drug dealer I had a product that could make people feel fantastic. As an acupuncturist it was as if I still had 'the gear' as I could create altered states in the client. Without drugs or acupuncture, I was now relying on a very different substance.

ENERGY FIELDS

This ability to shift people into altered states is connected with our energy field. In the seventeenth century, when it was discovered that two clocks placed together in a room would slowly synchronise their beat, it was termed 'entrainment'. The principles of entrainment are universal. They apply in chemistry, neurology, biology, pharmacology, medicine, astronomy and many other disciplines. They apply to spirituality as well. We all have energy fields, each with a certain vibration or frequency. When we are around others our energy fields align. The higher your vibration, the more powerful it is. Years of meditation and chi training make the vibration of your energy field so strong that others will synchronise with it. This is why you can feel euphoric and uplifted when you are in the presence of a spiritual master. Their energy field is vibrating so powerfully that it entrains your own energy field.

My twenty years of daily spiritual training, seeking a vibrational alignment with the source of highest good, enables me to use this potential in my work. I am no guru, but as a practitioner of traditional Chinese medicine, I know that the intention and life force of the healer influences the energy of the patient.[1] So I live in a way that constantly builds my life energy. Like Robyn, in the old days I woke up for drugs and went out scoring. In a way I still do this. The only thing that has changed is the substance. The new substance I want to score is derived from my daily spiritual practice of meditation, chi-building, weights and martial arts.

Living this way means that when the client arrives, higher vibrations from my daily practice are tangible. If my energy field vibrates at a frequency powerful enough to entrain the client's, they feel inspired and it assists healing to take place. The reverse is true too. As a youth worker, I had an energy field and organ system trashed from drugs. I was trying to help others while still craving drugs, bingeing on alcohol and marijuana, and feeling empty, depressed and lost. Being with clients then was hard because it didn't matter how much counselling took place, no one was progressing. Back then I didn't understand energy principles and I didn't know how to live, so we were all entraining each other in a negative way. It was a big mess. If you want to work with drug users, you've got to have something to give them apart from empty platitudes, guilt or more drugs.

If you want to work with drug users, you've got to have something to give them apart from empty platitudes, guilt or more drugs.

● ● ● ● ● ● ● ●

5 UNDERSTANDING PSYCHEDELIC EXPERIENCES

Psychedelic or hallucinogenic drugs are different to stimulants such as cocaine, speed or ice. Psychedelics are like the sharks of the drug world, predictable only in their unpredictability. Hallucinogenic trips can be mind-blowingly beautiful or hideous and terrifying. They can also instantly shift you into dimensions you are not prepared for, places where the rules of the normal world are not relevant and even fundamental physical laws such as gravity do not apply.

> Psychedelics are like the sharks of the drug world, predictable only in their unpredictability. Hallucinogenic trips can be mind-blowingly beautiful or hideous and terrifying. They can also instantly shift you into dimensions you are not prepared for, places where the rules of the normal world are not relevant and even fundamental physical laws such as gravity do not apply.

Stanislav Grof, a leader in the field of psychedelic therapy since the 1950s, once took a high dose of LSD and focused on projecting himself from a clinic in the US to his parents' home in Prague. He felt as if he really was in their home. Just as he started thinking of physically shifting something to prove that he had been there, he was overcome by terror. He had enough psychedelic experience to realise that if he confirmed what he had done, 'his whole universe would collapse'.[1]

On LSD you can be telepathic. You can bend the laws of time and space, interact with beings from astral realms, and communicate with plants. You can also shape the environment around you. Stephen Gaskin, a leading figure in the counter-culture, describes how one friend could take the spirit of what he was saying and make pictures of it for those with him. While Gaskin and this friend were on LSD, he talked about being 'outrageous'. As he said the word, he turned into a 'human-sized two-headed chicken with gold beaks, and lederhosen with embroidered suspenders. He was outrageous'.[2] These are good examples of a day in the psychedelic drug world.

With the current boom in recreational drug use, LSD or other psychedelic drug experiences are useful for any therapist working with drug users. A significant percentage of the population have used psychedelic drugs. Many have had experiences so far beyond the realms of reason that they are incomprehensible to a non-drug using person. I am not suggesting that health practitioners try mind-altering drugs, but there are many people in the industry who have had psychedelic drug experiences and whose insights could be drawn on as a resource. Psychedelic drugs open the doors to other worlds so the therapeutic approach needs to accept the concept of multi-dimensionality. If you have experienced this, you can more easily grasp the concept and the linked spiritual implications.

> I am not suggesting that health practitioners try mind-altering drugs, but there are many people in the industry who have had psychedelic drug experiences and whose insights could be drawn on as a resource.

LSD, SPIRITUALITY AND BAD TRIPS

Shortly after treating Robyn, I had a client, Melanie, a 26-year-old student who got more than she bargained for on a psychedelic trip. Melanie had often taken ecstasy with friends at dance parties and really loved the deep communal bond it created. When she was offered LSD, Melanie eagerly accepted. She was hoping that it would provide an opportunity for spiritual growth, and it did, but not in the way she had expected. On her trip Melanie had a revelation about the perfection of her own soul and the universe. It was so beautiful that she shed tears of joy. But at the peak of this experience a cold thought crept into her mind, that it was unnatural to feel so good, then panic set in. The trip turned bad. Fear, shock and dread replaced the euphoric bliss. She was surrounded by crazy, acid-coloured cartoonish imagery and was terrified she had lost her mind and would never recover.

The trip did end and Melanie's life did go back to normal. She forgot all about it until a few weeks later when, in a nightclub, the terrifying feeling came back. It overwhelmed her mentally and physically. This time she hadn't taken any drugs and couldn't shake it off. She thought she was going crazy and the fear of madness led to panic attacks. Melanie sought professional advice. Her psychiatrist assured her she was not mad, and said that she had an anxiety disorder. He offered her medication. But she didn't want more drugs, she wanted to know what was happening to her and why those feelings came back without the LSD.

UNFINISHED BUSINESS

As soon as Melanie started speaking, I saw she had 'reached for the Buddha state too soon'. Melanie chose the spiritually accelerating path of LSD and it had taken her where she wanted to go. When she entered this space, she was welcomed, but it was *she* who decided that she was not ready yet and rejected it. As the joy and euphoria welled up in her, Melanie felt like a thief, as if she had cheated on her soul. This was why the dark thoughts came in and the trip turned bad.

LSD magnifies *all* your feelings. It instantly intensified Melanie's sense of being unworthy. In my opinion it was an unfinished trip. If Melanie could recapture that state without drugs, and accept that she deserved it, she would be able to complete the journey the LSD started. Because Melanie took the drug seeking spiritual insight she now had to make it a *real* experience by committing to spiritual practice.

Hallucinogenic drugs such as magic mushrooms, peyote and ayahuasca have been linked to spiritual practices since ancient times. However, in that context they are never taken without physical and spiritual preparation. Melanie had not done any preparation. She wanted a powerful spiritual experience, but didn't realise the full implications of having it instantly delivered. In my interpretation of traditional Chinese medicine, the heart is the primary organ involved in hallucinogenic trips. The emotions and feelings associated with the heart are inspiration, love, shock and anxiety. The heart is also the seat of our spirit. This is why a psychedelic trip is either about bliss and sacredness, or shock and panic. Which way it goes depends entirely on how you respond to what is happening. This, in turn, is determined by the condition of your organs.

Melanie's pulse diagnosis revealed that, like many people of her generation, she had depleted organs, not so much from hard drug use but from lifestyle factors including no regular exercise and a nutrient-poor diet. Melanie's heart wasn't strong enough to allow her to feel self-love. Her kidneys were depleted, so she didn't have the capacity to forgive herself for not being pure, and she didn't have the will to accept the transcendent experience she was offered. Her spleen was also depleted, which meant she couldn't establish clear boundaries between herself and the new world she had entered, so she felt she was losing herself. Her spleen weakness also meant she couldn't mentally process what was happening, which contributed to her panic. Basically her organs were not able to provide the support required to experience the elevated state she had accessed. Hallucinogens also create a temporary separation of your body and mind (yin and yang). Your mind is set free but you need strong organs to enjoy this freedom otherwise the trip can turn bad.

With weak organs it is also hard to bring the mind back as you have no solid foundations to reconnect to reality. You feel your body is in one place and your mind in another, and anxiety and panic arise. After that trip Melanie did nothing to strengthen her organs, so the connection between mind and body remained fragile. The first panic attack happened at a dance party with pounding music and beams of light flickering over the crowd. This reminded her of the trip and triggered the panic and anxiety stored in her body. I recommended changes to her diet and

Hallucinogens create a temporary separation of your body and mind (yin and yang). Your mind is set free but you need strong organs to enjoy this freedom otherwise the trip can turn bad.

taking herbs and supplements, but also that she look into practices such as yoga to build organ strength, bring the mind back into the body, and introduce her to spirituality through physicality.

Melanie said that after that trip everything had been shaken to the core. What she had thought was real wasn't, and this was very frightening for her. I explained this wasn't necessarily a bad thing. Hallucinogens or psychedelic drugs made me understand there is more to the world than what we see. I learned it is only the inner journey in life that is important, and that there is definitely a spiritual aspect to existence. I have seen many clients like Melanie, people who have only one or two hallucinogenic trips but are changed for life. I wonder whether the soul planned this before incarnation, because it can create enough pain and chaos to force the person into self-development. If Melanie looked at the experience of her trip before it turned bad and aimed to recapture that, it would accelerate her spiritual development and change her life forever.

6 YOUR BODY TYPE AND FAMILY BAGGAGE

Marijuana changed my life and there is no doubt in my mind that it has contributed to a major shift in the way we think about each other, the environment and the planet. Like other drugs, marijuana can be an evolutionary tool on a global and individual level.

Nicki, a business executive, came for treatment for marijuana addiction. She was thirty-one and had been smoking since the age of sixteen. She had often tried to stop, but each time would end up going back to it and using even more than before. I could tell within minutes that she was what, in traditional Chinese medicine, we call a 'liver yang type', successful, driven and a high-achiever. She had a master's degree in business, had won medals in sporting competitions and was good at everything. She had naturally high energy levels and often had sex several times a day. Nicki was also a convert to the new age. She had lived in India, studied yoga and meditated regularly, but she needed marijuana every night and didn't understand why. She saw her marijuana use as a problem. Each time she smoked she was convinced she was taking a step backwards.

Marijuana was the little picture. Once Nicki understood the bigger picture, the nature of her relationship with marijuana, she would be able to make changes. Every drug plays a role in a person's life. If you give up without knowing what it is, it can remain unresolved and stop you progressing. Once you understand the role of a drug in your life and find something else to fulfil its function, you will be free to move on.

I began by asking Nicki about her family history. This is important in traditional Chinese medicine. We are not blank slates and the longevity and health of your family gives an indication of the life force you have inherited. I usually ask where the family comes from, what they do and how they live, to get an insight into the client's inherited weaknesses, strengths and gifts. There is the cultural energetic inheritance to consider as well. Generally speaking, with each cultural background comes an energetic quality and a specific diet that has developed over time to balance this quality. This needs to be taken into account when making lifestyle changes.

> Once you understand the role of a drug in your life and find something else to fulfil its function, you will be free to move on.

When I was at college and desperate to be a vegetarian, I had a consultation with a visiting professor of Chinese medicine who seemed to spend most of his time smoking cigarettes outside the classrooms with the students. When I told him I was trying to be vegetarian, he took my pulse, asked a few questions about my German heritage, then laughed and told me to eat meat as it would take about five generations for me to become vegetarian.

Nicki's family were of Polish and Russian extraction. They had been in successful businesses for generations. She had inherited their mental strength, which is an expansive form of energy. Nicki's parents had migrated when she was a child, but had kept their traditions and, like me, Nicki was brought up on a typical northern European diet high in meat and starch. Although she was not consciously aware of it, eating those foods made Nicki feel grounded. Once she embraced the new age, she became a vegetarian. She thought that meant just eating fruit, vegetables and raw foods, and forgot about a protein source. Protein is essential physically and emotionally. It provides the ground for emotional balance and development of yin. With her protein-deficient diet, Nicki's energy was no longer controlled. Unbeknown to her, the marijuana was fulfilling that function as, for Nicki, it had grounding (or yin) qualities. Marijuana can mask the symptoms of protein deficiency.

Nicki had never heard of such concepts, but found it made sense. Towards the end of each day she could feel a surge of energy moving through her that was difficult to control. She felt light-headed, agitated and nervy. The marijuana immediately took that sensation away, allowing her to feel calm and to meditate. She needed marijuana to follow her spiritual vision of being vegetarian, meditating and ultimately being a yoga teacher, because marijuana grounded her yang nature. So we had to find other means of doing this, then she could free herself from the marijuana and embrace the next step in her personal development.

Her diet was the most important thing to change. Diet is crucial for health in traditional Chinese medicine. Nicki really wanted to be a vegetarian, as this was recommended by her spiritual teacher and she didn't want to wait five generations to become one. But for westerners, being a vegetarian is more complex than just giving up meat and only eating vegetables. You have to be prepared to devote time and energy to making sure you have adequate protein intake. Nicki was also frequently experiencing diarrhoea from the raw foods, but if we introduced appropriate cooked foods and sources of protein it would improve this, and help ground her energy.

Another area to look at was her daily exercise. Nicki was doing yoga but it was a style that did not support her nature and energy. It is important to take up a form of exercise that supports your constitutional type, otherwise you can increase your imbalances. If Nicki studied a more athletic form of yoga or a martial arts style of exercise, it would allow her to express some of her energy but also help her understand her inner energetic forces and how to work with them.

While she was making these lifestyle changes, she could gradually start to reduce her use of marijuana. I suggested that instead of looking at the marijuana as a backwards step, she could look at it as having bought her the time to make the transition from her old lifestyle to a new one. She should consider it an evolutionary tool. It had allowed her to initiate important change within one generation rather than several. Nicki loved that idea.

When people work with their drug use from a new perspective, they can have powerful insights into themselves and their destiny. Looking back, all the insights I had with Robyn, about drugs allowing our true self to come forward, and with Melanie about how the hallucinogens show how much more there is to life than the material, also applied to me. But it wasn't until Nicki that I put all the pieces together. Marijuana had given her a chance to break with the old and move into the new.

BREAKING FAMILY PATTERNS

When I first discovered hashish I was still living at home. Each time I smoked I would have this recurring vision of an expansive landscape of green grass and blue sky. On one side was a hippie festival with lots of young people adorned with flowers, dancing and singing, and welcoming me with open arms. I longed to be with them and to experience their freedom. On the other side was my family, looking shocked and trying to get me to come back to them. I would always turn away from my family to the embracing arms

> I suggested that instead of looking at the marijuana as a backwards step, Nicki could look at it as having bought her the time to make the transition from her old lifestyle to a new one. She should consider it an evolutionary tool. It had allowed her to initiate important change within one generation rather than several.

> When people work with their drug use from a new perspective, they can have powerful insights into themselves and their destiny.

of the hippies. Letting go of my family was so blissful, tears would run down my face.

In session after session I work with my clients to show them how drugs allow them to consciously access the subconscious and how to retrieve that valuable information and work with it. Without my own past, I doubt I could have recognised these possibilities in drug experiences. Looking back, my own hash-vision had given me important information. I would see my family lined up, literally going back generations, and I had a strong sensation of not wanting to continue that line. My family was emotionally overbearing and at times violent. If I had joined that dynamic by being reactive and violent myself, I would have continued the pattern. I would never have been able to break free. Hash allowed me to break the chain, because I could separate from my family in a state of non-resistance. There was no big fight or confrontation, which would have triggered recriminations. I just drifted away.

Maybe I broke that chain forever. A long time ago I had a baby son who died at birth. It was the most devastating day of my life. I could never understand what had happened or why. I had no more children, so perhaps that chain is broken in more ways than one.

There was huge resistance within the family to my desire to be different. There would have been no support for me to break away from them, in this lifetime. At a subconscious level, drugs provided the support to get me through the first steps of that process. But I didn't realise it, so I kept using harder drugs. I became a lost soul. I didn't find myself again until I understood that I had to accept my family the way they were but at the same time live my life true to my spirit and my values. This is the way to evolve in accord with your soul's destiny.

PART II
GIVING UP DRUGS

7 HOW PEOPLE GIVE UP DRUGS

Taking up drugs is easy. Giving up is the hard part. While you are on drugs and having a good time, you don't think about quitting. That only happens when it all starts turning bad. As a result, giving up drugs is usually a hit and miss affair with a lot of unnecessary suffering. How we give up is influenced by the kind of person we are, but there is no easy way. Unless of course you give up at the beginning.

I could have taken the idea that my hash-induced vision of my family and the hippies was an important message from my subconscious and given up at seventeen. I was young, healthy and not dependent. It would have been so easy. My first fantastic LSD trip, around the same time, was probably another good time to stop. I saw how beautiful the world is and what an integral part of the cosmos we all are. That was it, the entire cosmic message delivered in one trip, but I didn't get it. I thought it was all about staying high on drugs.

Even now we know very little about altered states. Most people launch into drugs unprepared, then drift along. When I had my first taste of hashish I had no expectations, but I felt so unbelievably good that I wanted to do it again. It was the same when I tried LSD, cocaine, mescaline, magic mushrooms and speed. The only exception was heroin. I knew where doing that again would lead and didn't want to go there. Because I didn't understand drugs and didn't know my life's destiny, drugs became my destiny. They controlled me. This is what happens to many recreational drug users.

I have never met anyone who had a plan before they took up drugs. No one knows what they want from drugs, because until you go there you don't know what they offer. There are almost too many factors involved to predict what might happen. After seeing countless clients, I still can't find a logical explanation as to why some people repeat drug experiences and others don't. Or why some people become addicted and others don't, or why some people become psychotic or depressed and others don't. The only certainty in the drug world is that every drug user will have to give up one day. Recreational drug use is not permanent and all drug users know this. But because we don't understand drugs, we have no idea how to give them up.

> Because I didn't understand drugs and didn't know my life's destiny, drugs became my destiny. They controlled me. This is what happens to many recreational drug users.

> The only certainty in the drug world is that every drug user will have to give up one day. Recreational drug use is not permanent and all drug users know this. But because we don't understand drugs, we have no idea how to give them up.

For me, in the beginning, it was all so good I didn't want to stop. Later, when I became a speed addict, I couldn't stop. My drug use had gone way past recreational, and I knew it. I lived in squats with people in the same state as I was. Talking about giving up drugs was taboo. None of us could stop and we didn't want anyone around us to stop either. Drug-taking is not a solitary pursuit. Until the final stages of heavy addiction you generally want to be around people you can share that space with. You can instantly sense when someone in the group is moving away from drugs and you have to make sure they don't. You think that if they get clean they will reject you, then you will be alone.

I was not in an environment to support quitting, and I had no idea how to quit or what to expect if I did. Thirty years later nothing has changed. People repeatedly quit, then take up drugs again. Some hold out for weeks, months or even years before giving in. When I looked at how people gave up, I identified a couple of different methods: by willpower (the yang type termination), by love and support (the yin type termination), or by making a dramatic lifestyle change.

> Until the final stages of heavy addiction you generally want to be around people you can share that space with. You can instantly sense when someone in the group is moving away from drugs and you have to make sure they don't.

USING WILLPOWER TO QUIT

I have seen some clients who decide to give up drugs and do it on the spot. These are naturally strong-minded people, which is why this method can work for them. Lisa was a great example of this. She started smoking marijuana at fourteen. She always became highly paranoid, but as she was in a group of dope-smoking peers she continued anyway. Then she tried speed and things improved instantly. She loved it and would use speed while her friends smoked marijuana. This meant she could join in with them in an active and engaged manner rather than feeling like a zombie.

Speed introduced Lisa to the hard drug world, and she embraced it enthusiastically, using ketamine (an anaesthetic used in veterinary practice), cocaine, mushrooms, LSD, prescription medications and even whipped cream bulbs (she would buy packets and inhale the gas). She would frequently take herself to the frontiers of no return, and be 'brought back' by people frantically slapping her face and shouting her name.

By night Lisa dressed in patent leather, studded collars and chains. By day she was a business manager who wore conservative suits. She went to work every day, as most of my clients do, and managed all aspects of her life. Her drug use kept increasing though. When she discovered ice, she was instantly hooked. It wasn't long before she was using several grams a day. Then one morning she woke up, automatically reached for the ice before getting out of bed, and decided it had all gone too far. After years of serious substance abuse, she gave up that day. She still associated with her drug-using friends, but never touched drugs again.

Lisa didn't notice any immediate effects, except for finding herself with spare cash. She had no idea what to do with this and took to buying expensive handbags. Several weeks later, serious post-drug symptoms started. She felt confused, lost, paranoid, empty and alienated. The euphoria of giving up drugs had worn off and her true state of health was revealed.

USING THE SUPPORT OF OTHERS TO QUIT

Other people, yin types who are more passive, need someone else to help them to change. They feel they need the love, commitment or support of another person to fuel their drive to give up drugs. They look to their partner, or wait for someone to come into their life to play the role of helper or motivator.

Carl used speed a couple of times a week in controlled amounts. On weekends he would let go and binge. During one party weekend he fell madly in love with a beautiful, outgoing 21-year-old. She was attracted to him because he appeared to be a successful extrovert who loved to have a good time. She did not use drugs, but drank alcohol. They began to see each other regularly. Eventually her enthusiasm, spontaneity and passion for life made Carl think he was a fake, because he needed chemicals to be how she was naturally. Whenever he was with her it reminded him of how chemically dependent he had become. She unwittingly brought his drug problem to the surface and became the trigger for him to give up.

Carl decided that giving up drugs would be his mission, but believed he needed her to commit to him to give him the strength to fulfil this mission. She was young, however, and just wanted to have fun. She didn't want to hurt Carl so she kept avoiding the commitment issue. She was also not aware of the full extent of his drug use. She thought he was naturally outgoing, but this was an illusion created by the speed. Without drugs Carl was fragile, weak and introverted.

The relationship became messy. Carl tried to stop the drugs, but the pain of his girlfriend refusing to commit kept him going back to the speed. Eventually Carl saw her lack of commitment to him as the only thing stopping him from giving up, and he started to blame her for his habit. The relationship eventually broke up.

By then Carl had started the psychological battle to stop. Soon after he began a new relationship with a work colleague eight years older than him, who was a motherly type. She had been interested in him for a long time, but he had not reciprocated. She made a commitment to Carl and this empowered him to take the last steps. Their relationship ended after a few years, but he was finally drug-free.

DRAMATIC CHANGE IN LIFESTYLE

I have had many patients who started the process of giving up drugs by moving interstate, or getting jobs on fishing boats or oil rigs. Getting away from your peers and making big changes in what you do and where you are helps because its takes the focus off the drugs. It also provides an opportunity to redefine yourself without the pre-existing judgement of family or society. It is hard to quit when you are surrounded by people who don't believe you can, then say 'I told you so' each time you falter.

THE GOLDEN SHOT

Some choose to give up drugs with a deliberate overdose, or 'golden shot', because they cannot face the long and painful journey back from where they are. In general, the people who take this option have become chronically bitter about life. They never talk about suicide, but it is in their mind all the time. One day they look at the gear in front of them, put too much in the syringe and then think 'screw everything' and go all the way. This is far more common than people realise. If we

> It is hard to quit when you are surrounded by people who don't believe you can, then say 'I told you so' each time you falter.

understood how recreational drugs impact on the body, mind and spirit and if we knew we could recapture our passion and excitement in life after drugs, and be inspired to do so, the outcome could be different for so many people.

USING DRUGS TO FIGHT DRUGS

In many cases where people seek mainstream help, recreational drugs are replaced with pharmaceutical drugs. I regularly see patients who have given up illicit drugs but are on antidepressants, antipsychotics, sleeping pills, tranquillisers or, in the case of heroin addicts, methadone.

> If we understood how recreational drugs impact on the body, mind and spirit and if we knew we could recapture our passion and excitement in life after drugs, and be inspired to do so, the outcome could be different for so many people.

> The idea of using licit drugs to treat illicit drug addiction has been around for a long time, but from the perspective of traditional Chinese medicine, taking one type of mood-altering drug to counter the effects of another type of mood-altering drug is not a long-term solution.

The idea of using licit drugs to treat illicit drug addiction has been around for a long time, but from the perspective of traditional Chinese medicine, taking one type of mood-altering drug to counter the effects of another type of mood-altering drug is not a long-term solution. It might buy you some time and allow you to feel that change is possible, but *all* these drugs work by exploiting the resources of your organs. You may feel different for a while, but ultimately you will slowly feel worse.

As well as having no idea what they are doing with drugs, most people have no idea what drugs are doing to them. Before I studied traditional Chinese medicine, I was sure that my drug use had done irreversible damage to my brain. I had an image of this shrunken grey blob with holes in it like Swiss cheese. Western medicine was so fatalistic, I thought that I was permanently damaged. Discovering traditional Chinese medicine gave me hope. It made me realise I could rebuild my organs. It also explained all my weird post-drug feelings and offered a path back to health and limitless bliss.

Giving up drugs is the beginning, not the end. For too long everyone has focused solely on quitting drugs as the end goal. If you are a drug user, everyone wants you to stop. The government, health professionals, rehab centres, families and friends all think that if they can just get you to stop taking drugs, everything will be fine. It is this thinking that leads to constant relapse. However, if you look at giving up as the *beginning* of a journey, you have a much better chance of achieving success.

> If you look at giving up as the *beginning* of a journey, you have a much better chance of achieving success.

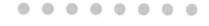

8 HOW NOT TO GIVE UP DRUGS

I saw giving up drugs as the end goal. By the time I wanted to stop, due to my excessive hard drug use I was neurotic and emotional, and didn't have the strength or the vision to give up on my own. Drugs were my whole world. All my friends and associates were drug users, and drugs were my business. Basically there wasn't much incentive to stop. I figured I was heading for the golden shot, and in the back of my mind had some vague idea of having as many highs as possible before that happened.

GIVING UP–THE INSPIRATION

It was a moment of inspiration and a dramatic change in location that kicked off my long drawn-out process of giving up. When I was still in Germany my family often talked about moving to Australia. Nothing in the straight world had any relevance for me but once they made the decision to leave, I was inspired by the idea of Australia. High on speed, pills and hashish, I had this vision of hitchhiking across the country dressed like a cowboy. I would meet farmers who would give me food in return for working on their farms. I'd sit around campfires at night, bonding with people and getting high on life, not drugs.

This vision gave me a momentary sense of a future, of hope, of the possibility of change. It made me remember how optimistic drugs used to make me feel. The idea of bonding with people based on love was what I had really wanted in life. I decided then and there to give up drugs. My reward for making this momentous decision was to drug myself into oblivion every day. With chemical hope coursing through my veins, everything looked easy. I left Germany and didn't return for nearly fifteen years.

I might have got the inspiration and the dramatic change in location part right, but nothing prepared me for the reality of quitting. By the time I arrived in Australia I was twenty-three and in really bad shape. Speed wasn't my only drug. I was regularly adding morphine pills, atropine (a poisonous alkaloid from deadly nightshade) and anything else I could get my hands on to get a high. The 'giving up' idea was still in my head, but I hadn't thought through the details.

I had brought a lot of powerful, high-quality prescription amphetamines with me and I had the vague idea that by the time I got through them, I'd have weaned myself off drugs slowly or found somewhere to score. It only took two days before I was down to my last handful of pills. I decided to end it with a bang. I met a couple of backpackers, amphetamine freaks like me, and we had a binge. We took the lot, and partied all day and night. It was paradise. The next day, my first day without speed, felt a bit strange but I was still riding on the memory of the previous high. By the second day my life had descended into chaos.

> I might have got the inspiration and the dramatic change in location part right, but nothing prepared me for the reality of quitting.

> The next day, my first day without speed, felt a bit strange but I was still riding on the memory of the previous high. By the second day my life had descended into chaos.

GIVING UP SPEED–DAY TWO

I was in a motel room in Sydney. Nausea, cramping and shaking convulsed my body.

There was a shrilling sound in my head that just wouldn't stop. I couldn't bear to look at anything because nothing made sense. My suitcase was lying on the floor, clothes spilling out of it. I wanted it all to be ordered but couldn't make it happen. There was a sock on the floor near my foot. I picked it up, then just stared at it. I had no idea why it was in my hand, or where it belonged. The shrilling in my ears now sounded like someone calling my name. I spun around but there was no one there. The voice was familiar, it was a woman I had met in Spain, but I couldn't work out why I couldn't see her, or why I was holding a sock. I realised I was part of some sort of game. It flashed into my mind that I shouldn't have gone to Spain. Suddenly I didn't know where I was, what country I was in, or what was happening. The internal pressure became unbearable. I had the urge to bang my head on the wall, so I did. Hard. The pain hit and in that moment of clarity everything made sense again. I wanted more of that pain-fuelled power. I wanted to destroy everything: smash the doors, windows, furniture, lamps, everything. I wanted to tear the place apart. It was the only way I could make things bearable. I got into it and started punching the wall.

A loud knock on the door made me stop. It was the manager, a middle-aged woman, asking what was going on. Realities shifted. I couldn't grasp what was happening. My knuckles were dusted with wall plaster and my forehead must have been red and swollen. I mumbled something about chasing a mouse. She got annoyed and said there were no mice. She looked at me like there was something wrong with me. I began to panic. I wanted to disappear because it was all too weird. I needed to prove that I was normal, so I said, 'But you've got a dog.' In my head this was a logical comment. I had seen a dog in the front office, and in my warped thinking dogs catch mice, so there must

> I wanted more of that pain-fuelled power.
> I wanted to destroy everything: smash the doors, windows, furniture, lamps, everything. I wanted to tear the place apart. It was the only way I could make things bearable. I got into it and started punching the wall.

● ● ● ● ● ● ●

have been mice. Now she looked at me like I was mad, and I realised I was losing my mind. She told me if I didn't stop she would call the police, then closed the door and left.

Confusion replaced my urge for pain. My brain was muddled and my head was spinning. I smoked ten cigarettes in a row to try and make sense of the chaos. I wanted speed so badly. It would put everything back into the correct boxes. Everything would be ordered and logical and then I would be able to relax. But I didn't have any.

SAYING YES TO PILLS AND ALCOHOL

I hadn't gone a day without speed for years for this very reason. I had no idea how long this was going to continue, or what would happen next. The only thing I knew was I couldn't stay still so I started hitching north

> I wanted speed so badly. It would put everything back into the correct boxes. Everything would be ordered and logical and then I would be able to relax.

to a hippie commune, numbing myself along the way with whatever medications I could get over the counter. Without speed and unable to smoke dope—because it made me so paranoid—I became dependent on pills. I took handfuls daily to control my symptoms.

This was where I started to use the 'replacement medication' model of giving up. But I wasn't under medical management and the way I took the stuff was dangerous and destructive. It wasn't enough either. I needed a kick, I needed speed. By the time I got to the commune any interest in getting high on life or bonding with farmers was gone. My life without drugs was unbearable. I was in a place where I couldn't get hard drugs, and this is the only reason I managed to stop taking them.

I was now on the opposite side of the world, away from my peers and out of the reach of hard drugs, but I felt so bad I just wanted to die. Then I discovered alcohol. The minute I realised lots of beer made my fear, introversion, depression, confusion and aggravation disappear, I became a committed drinker. Alcohol was a magic potion that allowed me to laugh and talk to people again. It didn't have the 'upper' buzz of speed, but at least I could interact socially and experience some positive feelings about life. Each night I would drink until I was unconscious. Alcohol allowed me to feel normal. The fact that I needed a couple of litres of it to reach that point really didn't seem like a problem compared to having needed speed to do the same previously. The hangovers were not as bad as speed hangovers, so it seemed a win-win solution.

> Alcohol allowed me to feel normal. The fact that I needed a couple of litres of it to reach that point really didn't seem like a problem compared to having needed speed to do the same previously.

By the time I had been free of hard drugs for nearly a year, I was pretty pleased with myself. The speed cravings were still there, but alcohol-fuelled crazy behaviour could get me through them. Then I became dependent on alcohol. It wasn't until I found myself craving it the way I craved speed that the penny dropped. But I had been medicating myself with various substances for so long that, instead of seeing this as a problem, I simply made sure that I never went anywhere without plenty of alcohol and pills.

After I left the commune, I moved to a ski town and found a job in the hospitality industry. The first night I headed off to the nearest hotel to drink myself unconscious. There was a live band playing and a huge crowd partying like there was no tomorrow. The atmosphere was electric. It was my first taste of serious nightlife since Germany and I desperately wanted to be part of it. I went to the bar to order a beer, but before I got there a lively-looking guy was at my side asking if I wanted speed. Unnerved and instantly stressed, I mumbled that I didn't do speed and he walked away. It was the first time in my life I'd said no to drugs. I felt really good. But seconds later I felt bad, because I had missed out. The party raged around me and everyone had a good time but me. It didn't seem fair.

SAYING YES TO DRUGS

It only took a few weeks for me to accidentally-on-purpose catch the eye of the dealer. As he walked towards me I knew the old battle was going to begin again, but I was so tired of the effort I thought, stuff everything, I'm going to do it, just for tonight, just one line to pep me up a bit. The moment I said yes, I felt so free it was extraordinary. I had been living in a world of pain, denial, suppression and cravings for so long it was an indescribable relief to stop fighting against everything and give in. I'd bought myself a ticket to paradise—I knew the next twenty-four hours were going to be awesome and I didn't care what happened after that.

It was the first time in my life I'd said no to drugs. I felt really good. But seconds later I felt bad, because I had missed out. The party raged around me and everyone had a good time but me. It didn't seem fair.

• • • • • • • •

As we walked outside to his car my anticipation and excitement built. I was high just at the thought of what was to come. He asked if I wanted a needle, but I said I'd snort it. I told myself that this would mean I was in control. He put out a line for me. The familiar bitter taste moved down the back of my throat and almost instantly a rush of euphoria, clarity, focus and energy flooded every cell in my body. I felt better than I had in years. I was back. It felt so good I did a second line. I thought it must have been really high-quality stuff, so I bought whatever he had left.

For the first time since I left Germany I was part of everything again. Instead of trying to hide from the world, I was outgoing, chatty and lively: the life of the party. It was miraculous, as though I'd been raised from the dead. The band was amazing, the crowd was on its feet, and it was an incredible night. The next three days were a speed-snorting extravaganza. Everything stayed fantastic until the drugs ran out.

It was mid-afternoon. I'd been awake for three days by that time and was exhausted, but my mind wouldn't stop. Then I had to go to my job in the kitchen. The orders in front of me made no sense. People were yelling at me but the sounds were echoing in my head. I was sure I was on the verge of collapse. It was a long time since I had felt that bad physically, but emotionally it was worse. Anger, shame and self-condemnation chased each other around in my head. I was weak, pathetic, a total loser and I just wanted to die. Nothing was worth feeling like this, so I swore to myself I would never do speed again.

Alcohol became my number one substance once more, but it couldn't deliver the results. It was only a matter of time before I gave in and got speed. This time I used a needle. I began using two or three times a week, and this kicked off a cycle of getting high, feeling disgusted with myself, giving up speed, then drinking in excess to control the speed cravings. Then, feeling contaminated, I'd try and be pure, and give everything up. That would be unbearable so I would end up bingeing again. At the same time I despised myself for my weakness and the cycle would start again. It was a horrible way to live, always desperately craving something and never being satisfied, never feeling good.

This is how not to give up drugs. Some things were right—getting away from my peers, making major lifestyle and location changes—but other things were seriously wrong. My biggest mistake was not replacing the drugs and alcohol with any other way to feel good.

My biggest mistake was not replacing the drugs and alcohol with any other way to feel good.

9 THE UNASKED QUESTIONS

My initial inspiration to quit occurred when I was in my early twenties but I had my last drug hit a good ten years after that. A huge percentage of current drug users have a similar experience. They no longer want to use drugs, but they just don't know how to stop. They don't know how drugs work, or when or how to give up. They also don't know why, or more importantly what, they are giving up. So, a lot of people who genuinely want to stop keep relapsing. Each time they go back to drugs they hate themselves.

Recreational drugs are a huge business but an illicit one. This means the information circulated about drugs focuses on prevention. Produced by non-drug users for non-drug users it has little impact on drug consumption. We need a deeper understanding of what drugs provide for people, and how to replace that. This means going into the forbidden territory of discussing drugs and pleasure. The truth is, drugs can make you feel so good it is almost incomprehensible, and everything after that seems dull and lifeless. But the rest of the truth is that we don't need drugs to feel that good. If someone had shown me back when I was a teenager why I used drugs, how they made me feel so good, then how to recapture what I wanted from drugs in other ways, everything could have been so different.

THE DISCOVERY PHASE

If you talk about how good drugs make you feel, you have to talk about how bad they make you feel, because the highs and lows are inseparable. Most drug journeys begin with the 'discovery phase', in which you learn new things about yourself, others and the universe. If you keep taking drugs the quality of the experience will eventually start to decline, so you try different drugs and larger doses. Sooner or later, though, you will reach the point where you can never recapture the intense excitement, joy or discovery of the early drug experiences.

When clients who were trying to quit came in, I began asking them to fill in a drug satisfaction graph. They had to mark the highs of the early days, and the highs they were getting at the end. They always drew a chart with a line that initially spiked then fell, and spiked and then fell. If you joined the high and low points, you got a big fat line descending straight down to the base. If you are taking drugs, ideally you want to pull out at the peak, at the beginning, then use those highs as the benchmark for how good you want to feel again in life after drugs.

> If you are taking drugs, ideally you want to pull out at the peak, at the beginning, then use those highs as the benchmark for how good you want to feel again in life after drugs.

● ● ● ● ● ● ● ●

THE MEDICINAL PHASE

While the transition from peak to trough depicts the inevitable outcome of ongoing drug use, it also reveals the shift from taking drugs to have a great time, to taking drugs to suppress side effects. Once you start on the decline, you will need drugs to control the symptoms of the drugs. The transition from taking drugs to feel good to taking drugs so that you don't feel bad is often so gradual that most people don't realise that it has happened. They think that maybe the drugs don't work as well or that the quality is poor. Looking for better drugs or mixing up different substances to try and recapture the highs can drag on for years. Once drug use becomes medicinal or habitual, your physical, emotional and mental health will decline. You will never recapture the highs, and will reach the point where you have to stop. Some take time out, get off drugs for a few months, then use drugs and get that discovery feeling again, but you can't hold it. It is temporary. Sooner or later it has to end.

ASKING THE RIGHT QUESTIONS

To give up drugs you need to ask the right questions. When clients say they want to quit drugs, I always ask why. This throws most people. Giving up is what every drug user is expected to do. No one asks why. But if you have been a long-term user and want to quit, you do need to understand why. Scores of clients say their partner, their family or parents want them to. If this is the main reason, it is not enough. You need to be clear about exactly why *you* want to give up— or, why you want to keep using. If you have a position you have something to work with.

Then there is the issue of *what* you are giving up. If you have been using daily, letting go of drugs can mean letting go of the most important thing in your life. Drugs structure your life and make it predictable. You know exactly what you are living for, and you find a way to get it. This gives you a strong direction. As soon as you stop, you won't have that anymore. Drugs can also play a support role by providing you with

The transition from taking drugs to feel good to taking drugs so that you don't feel bad is often so gradual that most people don't realise that it has happened.

Some take time out, get off drugs for a few months, then use drugs and get that discovery feeling again, but you can't hold it. It is temporary. Sooner or later it has to end.

If you have been using daily, letting go of drugs can mean letting go of the most important thing in your life. Drugs structure your life and make it predictable.

the energy to get through the day, or a sense of company and nurturing. They can also have a therapeutic aspect. So, if you are a regular drug user and want to give up, you need to figure out what role drugs play in your life, then work on getting a replacement plan in place.

I recently treated a fifteen-year-old girl, Tania, who smoked hydroponic marijuana every day after school, then spent hours immersed in the fantasy worlds of computer games. Her mother thought she was addicted to both, and desperately wanted her to stop, but every time Tania stopped she felt empty and depressed. Her mother had taken her to various health professionals who told her to stop using marijuana, then suggested she take antidepressants.

Tania is from the new generation of drug users, who have inherited the expanded awareness of the previous generation but have no means of expressing it. Fantasy games and drugs allow them this expression. One of the first things Tania said was, 'I can't give up drugs, I've just started.' She had discovered the world of altered states and did not want to stop. She hated everything else in her life, especially school. This is a common complaint. According to traditional Chinese medicine there is much more to life than the visible world. In fact the majority of the universe is hidden. Even in the west it is accepted that all known life, including the galaxies and stars, and school and everything else Tania hated, only constitutes a small percent of the universe. The remainder is composed of dark energy and dark matter. We still don't know what they are.

For Tania, the solution was interaction with the world beyond visible reality. We discussed what it was about marijuana that made life so good. She said 'being in a dream state, but being active'. I told her that drugs show but they don't create, and after drugs you have to create what you were shown. Tania immediately knew what I was talking about. So, we looked at permanent options for achieving that feeling of 'dream and action'. I explained that getting that feeling *without* drugs would require working with her organs, as they are the gateway to the invisible worlds. For her the place to start would be building up her life-force by working with her organs to produce altered states, just like drugs do. Most of the games Tania played were based on the art of war and fighting with supernatural powers, so I showed her images of the Shaolin monks performing extraordinary feats, and she was immediately fascinated and inspired.

HOW TO MAKE SOMEONE ELSE GIVE UP DRUGS

Her mother had hoped I would tell Tania to stop using marijuana, but everyone else had done that and it hadn't made any difference. Focusing on stopping drugs for Tania meant focusing on stopping something she wanted or needed. She didn't want to give up the journey the marijuana had started, but as I explained to her, she didn't have to—she could get to the same place by following a different path.

Telling someone to stop drugs does not work. Offering them another way to get what drugs provide is a better idea. All the people who wanted me to give up didn't have anything to offer me, apart from being like them, and I didn't want that. I wanted a wonderful, exciting and magical life. I didn't want to be bitter, cynical, stressed, reactive and living totally in the material, 'rational' world. Nothing about their lives was the least bit inspirational to me. If you want to help someone stop drugs, you have to have something the drug user wants. If you live in a way that brings magic into your life and a light into your eyes, if you are accepting of everything and everyone, energised and constantly discovering, expanding and exploring life, then you have something they want.

> Tania didn't want to give up the journey the marijuana had started, but as I explained to her, she didn't have to—she could get to the same place by following a different path.

> If you want to help someone stop drugs, you have to have something the drug user wants.

10 MARIJUANA, CHAOS AND ORDER

Tania was a great client. She wanted the magical feeling marijuana provided and because she had grasped the journey concept right away, and the idea that drugs show but don't create, she was open to other ways of continuing on that path. She also loved the Chinese ideas about the organs. As marijuana impacts primarily on the liver we talked about what a fascinating organ it was. The liver is connected with our dreams, but it is also the residence of the ethereal soul.[1]

The liver has a host of other functions including regulating the flow of life energy around the body. When chi flows freely, you feel happy. Marijuana enhances this function of the liver (explaining the fits of giggles it can trigger) but this is at a cost. Imbalances arise and eventually you get the exact opposite of what you wanted. Tania had only been using marijuana for a few months and was still feeling the positive emotions of her liver, but if she kept going, as so many people do with dope, the liver suffers, and happiness turns into irritability, frustration and bitterness. When people feel that way they tend to smoke more dope to take those feelings away. It is very hard to give up in these circumstances.

Another client, Susan, was also initially captivated by the magical quality of marijuana. Susan began smoking when she was seventeen and part of the surfing culture. She wore sarongs, was tanned and had long, bleached blond hair. She spent her twenties smoking marijuana with her friends and chilling out with reggae music. Dope was a key part of her lifestyle. She loved it but somewhere along the way it had run out of control. Twenty years later Susan was smoking thirty or forty pipes a day. She described her life as a mess, and felt scattered, directionless and lost. She knew dope was contributing to this on some level and had been unsuccessfully trying to give

> Tania had only been using marijuana for a few months and was still feeling the positive emotions of her liver, but if she kept going, as so many people do with dope, the liver suffers, and happiness turns into irritability, frustration and bitterness.

●   ●   ●   ●   ●   ●   ●   ●

it up for years. Every time she did, she felt frustrated and angry, and couldn't stop because she needed marijuana to control her anger.

Susan worked from home, running a T-shirt printing company, and had several casual staff. Her life was erratic. She got up at different times, worked different hours and ate meals randomly. Within this chaos the only constant was marijuana. She always knew how much dope she needed, and when she needed to score again, but her drug use was chaotic. Sometimes she would start the day with a joint, stay stoned until lunchtime, then work in the evenings. Other times it would be a completely different pattern. It depended on what she had on each day or how she felt.

The first thing Susan needed to do was to create order out of the chaos. Marijuana was the constant factor so we started with that. I explained that it was affecting her liver, the organ associated with movement, direction and happiness, but also frustration and anger. Initially she had been smoking to get that feeling of everything progressing smoothly in life and it delivered that, but because Susan had used marijuana for so long and had such an erratic lifestyle, she had major imbalances in her organs, including her liver, and that left her feeling frustrated and stuck. Every time she gave up she felt highly stressed and was liable to lash out at her staff. Marijuana gave her the feeling

Marijuana gave Susan the feeling of flow and movement but, unbeknown to her, it was slowly increasing her underlying frustration and anger.

● ● ● ● ● ● ● ●

of flow and movement but, unbeknown to her, it was slowly increasing her underlying frustration and anger.

Susan needed a plan to give up. I suggested that rather than focus on giving up, she instead had to focus on getting into a routine. She immediately rolled her eyes, because routine is the thing most drug users hate or resist. The boredom of doing the same thing day after day is one of the reasons people take drugs. Also, long-term drug users become scattered; trying to focus on one thing is uncomfortable. However, as I explained to Susan, it is less painful to create a routine than deal with the anger, frustration and confusion that arose each time she quit marijuana. She agreed.

As I outlined to her, routine means your life must be predictable. Everything must have its place from when you get up until you go to bed. Don't get up later than six each morning, have a bottle of water by the bed, drink it, then spend forty-five minutes doing some form of exercise. Walk on the beach, ride a bike down the street, anything. You can even begin by just sitting on the bed and staring at the floor. The idea is to try and get comfortable with the idea of spending time in your own company without cigarettes, joints, coffee, TV or radio.

This is going to be uncomfortable because once you have consumed a certain amount of drugs you lose your ability to be with yourself. The dope provides 'company'. If you want to give up drugs and have a happy and exciting life after drugs, beginning the day being with yourself is crucial. This space you establish in the morning is where you lay the foundation to recapture what the drugs have shown you, but without drugs. It is the first step to an awesome life after drugs.

After this sit down and have a wholesome, nurturing breakfast. Try cooked grains such as porridge, instead of processed breakfast cereals. If you usually smoke dope first thing in the morning, after breakfast you can have your first joint or a bong. Think of it as a reward for getting up early, drinking water, exercising and eating a wholesome breakfast. Always smoke dope *after* food, never before.

GIVING UP MARIJUANA

The next four hours, 8 am–12 noon should be an active time, with a snack around 10 am to help counter cravings—maybe have muesli or nuts. From 12 noon to 1 pm is lunchtime. Again, choose a wholesome cooked lunch, not sandwiches or cold food. Ideally you want protein, rice and vegetables. Then you can have marijuana again. This is the second session of the day. Break up the afternoon with a snack of fruit and nuts, then only have marijuana if you really need it to get the cravings down. Try and have dinner by 7 pm. Have a lighter version of your lunch menu. After dinner, it is time for a joint.

I wrote all of this down for Susan, then handed her the plan and suggested she try and follow it for six weeks, because that is how long it takes to create a habit. She was really surprised. She said she thought I was supposed to be telling her how to give up drugs, not how to take drugs. I told her that, in the situation she was in, to give up she first needed to be in control of it. Being in control means knowing where drugs belong in your life and what role they play.

Susan had never had any routine in her life and getting a system in place was really hard at first. But her chaotic life had become unbearable for her. She was no longer enjoying dope or anything else and wanted change. She started to create order in her drug use and lifestyle. Most importantly, she got the foundation in place for 'replacement' by getting up early and having that time with herself. It took her about five weeks with frequent lapses, but she constantly reminded herself that not doing this would ultimately make life more difficult.

> Being in control means knowing where drugs belong in your life and what role they play.

Because there were set times in place to use dope, after eight weeks on this program, Susan had managed to reduce her intake from thirty bongs a day to ten on weekdays and fifteen on weekends. This meant that she had times of clarity, followed by periods when she was stoned. For the first time in years she could distinguish between the two states. She had established a new rhythm so she felt stronger in herself, and had got to the point of having a short run along the beach in the morning. Susan's frustration was lifting because she had glimpses of her life improving. This feeling of natural improvement is a hugely addictive experience, more addictive than drugs.

> Susan's frustration was lifting because she had glimpses of her life improving. This feeling of natural improvement is a hugely addictive experience, more addictive than drugs.

● ● ● ● ● ● ●

In our next session Susan was enthused and inspired, and asked if she should give up completely now. But she had been smoking for over twenty years, and I knew that giving up at this point would be too dramatic for her. I suggested she reduce her intake again by fifty to seventy percent (three to five on a weekday and five to seven on Saturday and Sunday). The next step would be to continue the routine, but now look at the 'therapeutic' role the marijuana was playing. Susan had started smoking dope to feel mellow and at peace with nature and people, but her long-term use had damaged her liver and other organs, making her an angry, aggravated person. As marijuana use was simultaneously contributing to and managing these symptoms, we had to establish an alternative method of correcting her underlying imbalance. I suggested a program of weekly acupuncture and Chinese raw herbs.

On her next visit, Susan felt even better. Again, she wanted to stop completely. I told her that now was the time to focus on not doing breakfast bongs. If that felt fine, the next step would be to try and not smoke until lunchtime. When she got comfortable with that, she could drop the afternoon dose for a couple of weeks. The long-term aim was to only smoke marijuana in the evening after dinner. While she went through that reduction process, the focus would be on really developing her morning routine. Every time she reduced her marijuana intake, she had to add something to her morning routine. This could be some stretching or endurance training. The aim is to replace the actions of the marijuana. Stretching does this by engaging the liver and developing liver yin qualities (the qualities of marijuana). By the time she was having just one bong at night, her morning routine should be around an hour.

Over time this routine, the improved diet, Chinese herbs and rhythm in life would keep building Susan's inner energy levels, organs and emotional balance. Feeling mellow and peaceful would then come from within rather than from marijuana, and she would no longer need it or miss it when it was gone.

11 MARIJUANA AND ADDICTION

Marijuana is a paradoxical and complex drug. For many clients like Susan it begins as a way to chill out and have a laugh with friends, but then due to its impact on the liver, it takes on a more therapeutic role. The liver is unique amongst your organs. It has a dual function. The liver yang function, known as 'advance and act', allows you to move forward in life, while the liver yin function of 'retreat and wait' allows you to sit back. As a hallucinogen, marijuana has a magnifying effect and can enhance these very different functions.

My next client after Susan was Simon, a lawyer who had a highly stressful job. Each morning he had to face a desk laden with files needing urgent attention. These files represented people's lives, and the responsibility of that overwhelmed Simon. He was overloaded with work and had no idea where to start. He usually began by having a joint, and was then able to work methodically through the pile. He smoked marijuana at regular intervals throughout the day. He thought everything was fine but his wife thought he was addicted, and kept trying to get him to quit. Nothing worked and she finally threatened to leave him.

Simon agreed to quit that weekend. Monday morning he looked at his desk and felt like screaming. Without marijuana his aggravation escalated through the day. Everyone was moving too slowly. Everyone was in his way, so he yelled at all his staff. On the way to court the drivers around him were crawling along and he had to restrain himself from getting out of the car and punching someone. By Wednesday afternoon he had half his staff in tears, and files were piling up. He couldn't stand it anymore, so he had a joint and things immediately went smoothly again. The following day he reverted to his old habit, but his wife started urging him to quit again. A new pattern began: Simon would give up but then become so aggravated and aggressive he would take it up again. Eventually his staff refused to work with him unless he was smoking dope, so he was caught between his career and his wife.

His wife booked him in to see me. I did pulse and tongue diagnostics, and instantly identified a strong liver yang type. That quality can be a huge asset in life, as it is an important ingredient for business success, but it can also turn into your enemy if it is not understood and balanced by yin qualities. Simon had no balance in his life. He worked six or seven days a week, ate on the run and hardly slept. The yang ran out of control, which was why he moved much faster than his environment. Accordingly, he was constantly aggravated by people 'blocking' him. While marijuana made life chaotic for some people, it did the opposite in Simon's case. It gave him a sense of space and also allowed him to handle the slow speed everyone else worked at.

THE LIVER AND HOW WE EXPERIENCE TIME

The liver is the organ responsible for movement and it is also directly connected with our perception of time. Marijuana temporarily enhances the 'retreat and wait' function of the liver, so when you smoke marijuana, everything slows down. For liver yang types, such as Simon, who move faster than most people, smoking dope can enable them to accept a slower pace. This can work the other way as well. For many long-term dope smokers who don't have that natural drive and energy, the yin becomes so dominant that all they can do is retreat and wait.

I suggested that Simon not worry about giving up dope yet, but instead implement strategies to create a sense of space and time again. There are some very effective Chinese raw herbs that have an almost sedative quality, and certain acupuncture points can create a sensation of having space and time. In addition, a program of tai-chi, which works with your inner energy flow, would help Simon understand his nature and how to balance his yang without marijuana. Once he felt he could tolerate a slower pace, he could progressively reduce the dope. As marijuana had become medicinal for him, like a prescription medication, he needed to follow rules when he was getting off it.

MEDICINAL MARIJUANA

A lot of people end up self-medicating with marijuana without realising it. Karin came to see me because she had just given up dope but was feeling so bad she was thinking about taking it up again. Karin had used marijuana regularly for fifteen years, and was worried she had become dependent, so she quit. Instead of feeling better, she felt emotionally weak, vulnerable and exposed. She couldn't stand to be in a confined space with her husband and couldn't understand why.

> A lot of people end up self-medicating with marijuana without realising it.

In the consultation I took her back to the first joint she had, and how it made her feel. She said she was about thirteen, and as soon as she smoked marijuana she knew it was what she needed. It made her feel right. Karin had not mentioned happiness, laughter or magic as some people do when describing their early marijuana experiences. This was an indication that marijuana was something more than fun for her. I asked more questions about how her life was at the time. It emerged that she had a childhood of prolonged abuse and neglect. For as long as she could remember she had lived in fear. At the age of four she was sexually abused by her father, a violent drunk, and by an uncle. The abuse continued regularly. Her mother was often unconscious from alcohol, drugs or violence. Her only sibling had sided with their parents. No one had ever cooked her regular meals or provided any warmth, nurturing or routine.

In traditional Chinese medicine terms, she had no opportunity to develop the healthy yin energies that enable you to sit back and relax. During her childhood Karin had been consumed by anger and hatred of her father and uncle. She constantly fantasised about killing them and getting revenge. As marijuana is primarily a yin drug, as soon as she had that first joint, she could temporarily relax and let go. The dope also suppressed her desire for vengeance. If you look at your past in a state of yin you can forgive. If you lack yin you can be trapped in anger and rage. The more yin qualities you establish, the more you can control your anger and resentment towards others.

Karin's use of marijuana had been therapeutic rather than recreational right from the start. So when she gave up, all her physical, emotional and spiritual imbalances resurfaced. Emotionally she felt vulnerable and confused because a lack of yin leads to irritability, depression and anxiety. Physically she ached and kept tearing muscles, because yin is also responsible for lubrication of the muscles and tendons. So the key factor in her wellbeing was to build up yin by resting, eating correctly and sleeping regularly. To build up yin you also need adequate protein intake, supplements, medicinal herbs and a technique, such as meditation, that allows you to go within.

A major issue for Karin was going to be facing her history of abuse, but that would come later. If you want to examine your painful past, your organs have to be up to it first, otherwise you won't have anything to 'hold on to' when you are facing terrible memories. It is essential to develop strength

> Karin's use of marijuana had been therapeutic rather than recreational right from the start. So when she gave up, all her physical, emotional and spiritual imbalances resurfaced.
>
> If you want to examine your painful past, your organs have to be up to it first, otherwise you won't have anything to 'hold on to' when you are facing terrible memories. It is essential to develop strength prior to processing pain.

prior to processing pain. I wish I had known this when I was in youth work. We were supposed to get the kids off drugs, then make them sit and talk about things that were so excruciatingly painful, most healthy people wouldn't have been able to deal with them, let alone someone whose organs were damaged from deprivation and drug use. Confronting your past without enough physical strength can trap you in unbearable pain.

I worked out a program for Karin that included high-powered nutritional supplements and Chinese raw herbs. I also introduced her to my chi-conscious weight training exercises to target specific organs and muscle groups to build self-worth, strength and flexibility, the essential tools for facing and processing pain.

MARIJUANA AND LIFESTYLE

I frequently treat people who want to quit because they think they have become addicted to marijuana. Most can't understand why, as marijuana is not usually considered to be addictive—compared to heroin, speed or painkillers. In many cases it is not marijuana that is the problem, but the person's lifestyle.

At one time I treated quite a few tradesmen for marijuana addiction. One client, Tim, would get up at 5 am, grab a can of cola and drink it in the truck on the way to work along with smoking a couple of joints. The marijuana, caffeine and sugar provided a sense of energy, so he was not hungry. When he got to work he would have another joint while contemplating his tasks for the day.

Tim would have a couple of coffees and more marijuana in his morning break, then have nothing, or an occasional meat pie with a few more cans of soft drink, for lunch. This was followed by more joints. He was able to 'power' through the day until around three in the afternoon when he finished work. By the time he drove home he would be feeling really aggravated and uncomfortable. When he got home he sat on his deck drinking beer and smoking dope to unwind. He had no motivation to cook dinner for himself and would order pizza or other take-away food.

Tim had started this lifestyle as an apprentice when he was around seventeen. He had no idea it was having any negative effect, so he had no reason to change. But after twenty years this lifestyle had started to take a toll. His frustration kept increasing so that he needed more dope through the day to enable him to handle situations without losing his temper. He regularly had road rage, which got so bad that one day he ran someone off the road. It turned out to be an off-duty policeman and Tim was lucky not to have ended up in jail. Marijuana alleviated his frustration, so he smoked more to avoid the road rage. Tim worried he was getting addicted, so he quit, but then he was unable to control his frustration and anger, and he would suffer severe insomnia as well.

We need a healthy level of yin to be able to fall asleep. As Tim was yin deficient he needed marijuana to fulfil this function as well. Each time he quit dope, he would last about a week without sleep and days of frustration and anger, before it became unbearable and in desperation he would use marijuana again. He took this to mean he was addicted, but in his case the underlying symptoms were primarily to do with his lifestyle. The ongoing depletion of his organs due to poor diet and excessive sugar and caffeine intake had been damaging his yin. He needed the dope, the yin drug, to manage this—it was controlling and masking the symptoms.

Tim's yang constitution, without the yin to balance it, also affected his sex-life. The imbalance between yin and yang created 'heat', which he felt as a sexual itch. He would ejaculate three times a day to take the 'edge off' this uncomfortable condition. Excessive sexual activity is not beneficial as too much sex depletes the life essence stored in the kidneys (jing). This can lead to sexual

> The imbalance between yin and yang created 'heat', which he felt as a sexual itch. Tim would ejaculate three times a day to take the 'edge off' this uncomfortable condition. Excessive sexual activity is not beneficial as too much sex depletes the life essence stored in the kidneys (jing). This can lead to sexual dysfunction in later life.

dysfunction in later life. I suggested Tim reduce his ejaculation to once a day if possible, but the main focus was on making dietary changes. Food creates life. The more intelligence you apply to what you eat, the more effectively you prepare the ground for emotional, physical and spiritual wellbeing, and the less you will need drugs to create the impression of wellbeing.

Like many of my clients, Tim had simply never thought about his food before. It was just something to fill his stomach. Once he did, he really got into it. He took classes in Asian cuisine, bought an electric wok and started cooking his own lunch on the building site. His workmates initially ribbed him but then they started bringing in ingredients and asking him to cook them lunch as well. Tim replaced some of his cans of soft drink with mineral water, and implemented the 'dope as reward' system. He also had regular acupuncture, deep tissue massage and Chinese herbs. I didn't hear from him for a while until, a couple of months after our last session, I got a text message from him: 'You bastard, I forgot to smoke today.' And that was it. He never smoked dope again.

12 UNDERSTANDING SPEED

Each person's drug use has its own challenges and characteristics. Once you identify them, the way forward is more apparent.

Bob looked like a professional footballer. He had the large-framed body, the designer T-shirt, the jeans and gold chains. He had been a heavy speed and hard-drug user for several years, had been through rehab several times, but always went back to drugs. He had just come out of rehab again, and this time he wanted to make it hold, otherwise his wife was going to leave him and take the kids. He was a strong character physically and mentally, and I knew it was going to be a challenging case.

I asked Bob what happened in rehab. He said it was all fine except for the fact that they seemed obsessed with finding out what had gone wrong in his life to make him take drugs. Nothing had gone wrong. He had a great childhood, great family, lovely wife and terrific job. The other problem with rehab was that he refused to feel guilty or ashamed of what he had done—he loved drugs. They were pure adrenalin. He spoke openly in rehab about this and caused conflict, as you are not allowed to love drugs. You are supposed to be remorseful.

He would get off drugs in rehab, but once home the cravings were the big problem. They would be so powerful that he would use drugs again. The rehab centres suggested he look at pictures of his children to override his urge to use. Bob would look at pictures of them and feel love, but it had no impact on his cravings.

PLAYING BY DIFFERENT RULES

When it comes to drugs like ice and speed, you are up against such a powerful force that you need something stronger than the parenting instinct to counter it. Only a non-drug user could consider the love of your children as powerful enough to counter hard-drug cravings, because that is probably one of the most powerful forces in their lives. They don't understand the nature of the relationship that can develop between a drug and an addict. The drug becomes synonymous with your life force. For some people the attraction to drugs goes even deeper than human bonds. You are no longer operating by the rules of the normal world, so your emotional and ethical outlook is not comparable to that of a non-drug user.

For some people the attraction to drugs goes even deeper than human bonds.

● ● ● ● ● ● ●

I had another client recently, a pretty 22-year-old stripper who got an incredible rush from the power she felt over the men in the audience. In the nightclub environment she was constantly exposed to drugs, and eventually started using speed. This intensified her sense of power ten times over. Her speed use eventually led to heroin addiction. Needing more money, she became a sex worker. Her parents were devastated. They were a nice suburban Catholic family and had no understanding of what was happening. One day her father broke down in tears asking me how his daughter could do this to them.

In traditional Chinese medicine, drug use impacts upon all the organs. The heart is the organ that houses the mind and is the seat of judgement. Once its function is impaired you no longer have the judgement, ethics or morals of a non-drug user. You don't feel anything when you sell your body, take your parents' television, or use your kids' Christmas money to score drugs. This behaviour arises from organ dysfunction and is not intended to hurt anyone. You simply do not have the facility for judgement. This is why you feel no remorse.

YOU CAN'T SUPPRESS WHAT EXCITES YOU

Bob was my first client who openly claimed to love drugs and to have no regrets about his drug-taking. Drugs were his passion and his business, as he was a speed cook and dealer. This created another problem for him in rehab because it always offered such

> The heart is the organ that houses the mind and is the seat of judgement. Once its function is impaired you no longer have the judgement, ethics or morals of a non-drug user. You don't feel anything when you sell your body, take your parents' television, or use your kids' Christmas money to score drugs.

a great opportunity to liaise with other cooks, dealers, suppliers and users. The urge to do business was irresistible. During his second last stint in rehab, Bob had put a new team together and had produced a batch of speed. He said he just couldn't resist the challenge, it was exciting, and it was what he did.

He loved converting different chemicals into speed, then converting that into money. He would spend months in libraries studying chemistry and working out how to access the chemicals he needed. He probably knew more about chemistry than most qualified chemists. He said half seriously that he often thought of going straight and becoming a chemist.

The problem for Bob was that as soon as he produced drugs, he would start using again. In the end he and his associates would use more than they sold. They would become scattered, business went bad, money started going and Bob would end up in rehab. He always knew how it would end, but couldn't stop himself doing it, because he felt so good on speed or ice. For him, cooking and dealing was living life to the full.

CHASING THE BUZZ

I could relate to this. I still remember the buzz of successfully getting across a border or through customs with gear on me. The thrill is indescribable. You are right there, living in the moment, there is nothing else. You need to do it again.

I asked Bob what else gave him a rush. He thought for a while. He had tried skydiving and white-water rafting, but found them boring. Then he remembered doing kick-boxing in his youth, which gave him a real buzz. I told him we would make a list of exactly what excited him. It was fighting, fitness, dealing and using. We looked at the list and I said, 'Well, from your list, it looks like jail could be a good career option.' He laughed. I asked him what else would go on the list and he said 'freedom'. He really loved his children too, so we added them as well.

So, what excited Bob was fighting, fitness, freedom, his family and enhanced states. I suggested he had to make his life revolve around those qualities via a non-destructive, legal method. The only way to do this was through self-realisation, of building body, mind and spirit, in accord with what he loved.

First we had to tackle his symptoms. Bob had lower back pain, sore knees, tinnitus, frequent urination, dry retching after food, stomach cramps, no appetite, cravings for sweets, dizziness, blurred vision and no sex drive. He couldn't focus on one spot as it made him uneasy and nauseous. He also felt irritated, anxious and frustrated, and had shortness of breath, a wandering mind and chest pains. He could only stay awake for a few hours at a time. I suggested Chinese herbs and supplements to start relieving these symptoms and to help counter cravings. Bob said he was already taking vitamin B but it wasn't making any difference. I explained that just as there is a difference between good and bad speed, there is a difference between effective and non-effective supplementation. I work with the new generation of supplements, the relaxants, tonifiers and energisers based on Chinese herbal remedies, and powerful superfoods high in antioxidants. These treat emotional as well as physical symptoms.

SPEED, SEX AND LIBIDO

Since Bob had left rehab he had no desire for sex. It is common to have serious loss of libido after extended drug use, due to kidney depletion. It does not take long to correct with Chinese raw herbs and supplements. I have had clients who lost their sex drive, then developed a fear of having sex, which contributed to their inability to hold an erection. In most cases they returned to normal within weeks of treatment. It depends on what drug they used, and for how long, as well as other factors, but in traditional Chinese medicine it can be remedied.

Bob followed all my advice and on his next visit felt physically a bit better, although he was still feeling off and 'hanging out for a shot'. I asked him to describe his hanging-out feeling. I sensed something wasn't right here. He said he found it extremely difficult to be alone, because the temptation to use speed was so overwhelming. Whenever he was in the car he had to battle a force as strong as gravity pulling him to a dealer's house. As he talked more, it turned out that not only had Bob given up speed and ice, but also cigarettes, marijuana and alcohol.

He was expecting me to be impressed, but the warning lights flashed. Giving up drugs is the start of a lifelong journey, and it requires time and planning. I knew if Bob continued down the path of total abstinence he would be back on the rehab circuit in no time. Rather than congratulating him, I told him, 'You're going too fast, you will crash.' I suggested he keep smoking cigarettes and a little dope while we worked on building strength and health. He said if he did that, his family would think he was addicted to

It is common to have serious loss of libido after extended drug use, due to kidney depletion. It does not take long to correct with Chinese raw herbs and supplements.

Giving up drugs is the start of a lifelong journey, and it requires time and planning. I knew if Bob continued down the path of total abstinence he would be back on the rehab circuit in no time.

dope. I pointed out that surely that was progress compared to being addicted to speed. He looked a bit surprised, then agreed.

The side-effects of dope are nowhere near as bad as speed. Speed is a bastard of a drug. The confusion, the edginess, the urge for violence and the lack of focus make coming off speed torture. Some of my clients say it's worse than getting off heroin. With heroin at least you have physical symptoms you can grasp, but with speed you can't grasp anything, and it seems to go on forever.

THE WAY FORWARD

By the third session Bob's physical symptoms were under control. Bob said the treatment was working, that I had really helped him and everything would be different now. He had even driven past a dealer's place without feeling cravings or sadness. His parents and family were happy to welcome him back as a functional member of society. He looked at me waiting for me to acknowledge that I had done a good job, but I resisted. Therapy can quickly go into game playing, particularly in the drug world where people live by different rules. They understand what they need to say and do to keep things going in the direction that suits them.

I had learned this the hard way. Back in the eighties when I was working with the street kids I had been counselling a particularly violent and angry youth for about six weeks. He seemed to be able to relate to me and I was guiding him through a process of moving away from his violent behaviour and abuse of drugs into a more healthy way of living. We were really gaining ground fast and his ongoing positive changes were lifting my self-esteem.

Then one Friday afternoon he showed up in my office for his usual session. He shut the door and gave me the coldest look

> Therapy can quickly go into game playing, particularly in the drug world where people live by different rules. They understand what they need to say and do to keep things going in the direction that suits them.

I had ever seen. He told me I was a stupid fucking idiot, and did I really think I had helped him, did I really think I was helping anyone? He said that all along he had been playing me and he and his friends pissed themselves laughing about me. He told me that I hadn't changed him and never would, that I knew nothing about him. Then he leant over the desk, grabbed my throat and told me that if I even came near him again he would kill me.

Heavy drug users are so accustomed to being judged and so desperate to be accepted, they are going to look for emotional responses to their actions from their therapist. As soon as Bob started telling me how I had helped him, I knew he was waiting for me to establish a position as the successful, helpful therapist and to feel good about myself. I remained totally neutral.

He looked me straight in the eye and said, 'Any second this could collapse.' I still didn't respond. I knew he was waiting for me to take the next position of concern or compassion. When I didn't fall into the 'how can we avoid this?' trap, he made the third pass and said, 'I know I will use again, it's just a matter of time.' He was making the point of telling me that as soon as he felt physically better, he was going to use again.

I nodded and said in a matter-of-fact tone, 'Speed is a wonderful drug, of course you will.' Now he didn't know what to say. I told him that just because he had a few symptoms easing off didn't mean things had changed. All he had done so far was to start to repair the organ imbalances that the drugs had created; we hadn't addressed the real problem yet. Once he had had such extraordinary drug experiences and all this excitement, the memory was there for life. If he didn't find something to match it, he was always going to be tempted back to drugs.

But, I pointed out, drugs are temporary. Each time you use a drug like speed or ice, it reduces the quality of your next experience. I told Bob how I had once gone to a dealer in Amsterdam who gave me a really pure line of speed, but I had used so much by then that it tasted dirty or cut. I complained and the guy threatened to throw me in a canal. My system was too depleted to register a clean high.

Bob knew what I was talking about. Honestly, the only reason he went through rehab was to build up his health so that when he got out, the drugs would feel good again. I hear this all the time from people who use rehab as a break to rebuild for the next round. That approach too has a limited life. What is needed is to recapture the feeling, the intensity and exhilaration of the drug experience, and this is where the invisible worlds come in to the picture. The doorway to those worlds is via building chi or life energy. Because Bob loved fighting and had some more energy now, I suggested he take up kung-fu.

The next time he came in he started by telling me his best friend, also an addict, had come over with speed for Bob. For twenty years he and his friend had shared amazing experiences on drugs. They had a strong bond. The friend was now sensing that Bob was losing interest in drugs, that serious change was taking place, and this was making him feel vulnerable and scared.

Bob had looked at the speed but had no interest in taking it. This was the first time in twenty years he had no interest in drugs. He couldn't believe it. He was expecting me to say how great that was, but once again I took no position. I don't ever take a position because then the client knows I'm not judging them either way. Whether they are on or off drugs it doesn't matter to me. The client has to know that what they are doing is not for the therapist. Showing you are pleased with a client's progress means that if they do relapse, they will fear rejection and may not allow you back in their space. To work effectively you need to operate in an area where acceptance or

> What is needed is to recapture the feeling, the intensity and exhilaration of the drug experience, and this is where the invisible worlds come in to the picture. The doorway to those worlds is via building chi or life energy.

> I don't ever take a position because then the client knows I'm not judging them either way. Whether they are on or off drugs it doesn't matter to me. The client has to know that what they are doing is not for the therapist.

rejection are not issues. You want a blank slate. Whatever decision the client has made, the therapist will meet them there and have a creative response ready.

Instead I said, 'So, what excites you now?' Bob thought for a while then said, 'Nothing really.' This was dangerous territory. He was riding on the novelty of being drug-free, which is a kind of high. His cravings were under control because of the supplements, herbs and acupuncture but, as I knew from my own experience, once all that wore off he would feel empty. He had to get emotionally involved with something fast. I asked what his first thought was when he saw the speed. He said he felt sorry for his friend.

This was an indication that profound changes were occurring. When Bob looked at the drugs his first thought wasn't about himself, but about his friend. If he was still hooked his first thought would have been about himself. So I asked, 'How do you feel about your friend?' and Bob said he would love to get him off drugs. I knew immediately this could be a powerful force to drive Bob forward. Ex-drug users who rebuild themselves, and recapture what they wanted from drugs without drugs, feel inspired and are inspirational to others around them. I told Bob the only way to get his friend to change would be to inspire him by example. This meant his life had to be as charged-up, exciting and fulfilled as it had been on speed and ice.

Bob was a classic example of someone not interested in conformity. Part of the excitement for him was living outside the square. If he gave up drugs without finding a way of continuing to do that, as he had done the last seven times, it meant going back to drugs. I kept thinking about how Bob had jokingly said he might become a chemist. I don't think he would have lasted very long at that, but it suddenly struck me that he should become an alchemist. I told him that as a speed cook, he had turned base chemicals into financial gold and he produced magical substances to

> Ex-drug users who rebuild themselves, and recapture what they wanted from drugs without drugs, feel inspired and are inspirational to others around them.

transform people's consciousness. Alchemy was his passion, so this was the path to continue on, but he had to change the substances he worked with. He had to get into the Chinese martial and healing arts and experience the transformational potential of the body, the magic of the organs and then inspire others to do likewise. Helping people in this way resonates with the heart, and your deepest soul purpose. It can be a very addictive experience.

Bob needed to do kung-fu not to fight, but to transform. I also talked to him about Dim Mak, the ancient art of striking points on the body which can cause such damage to the internal energy system that your opponent dies. However, many of these pressure points also have great healing power. The theories of how to harm and how to heal are intertwined. All of this fighting, healing and transformative knowledge is incorporated into traditional Chinese medicine. Bob was really taken by all of this and signed up for some private lessons in the alchemy of Chinese medicine.

PART III:

HOW NOT TO LIVE
AFTER DRUGS

13 SAYING YES, AGAIN

I wish, when I was giving up speed, I could have said to myself everything I said to Bob—particularly identifying what I loved about it and replacing that with something other than alcohol or pills, but also about remaining true to myself. What I liked about Bob was that he loved drugs and the business. He knew who he was and refused to feel guilty for anything. In the first few years after I quit drugs I had no idea who I was so I worked hard to appear to be like everyone else. My biggest fear while on drugs was to end up living a boring nine-to-five existence, to not be free. But, for some bizarre reason that is exactly the life I set up for myself. I pretended to be straight. I turned into my own worst nightmare.

Secretly, I still wanted a non-conforming psychedelic life, but with no role models who had come out the other side of hard drugs, honest about their past and energised, passionate and still living each day as if life was a great adventure, I had no idea I could aim for such a thing, so I gave up. My life after drugs was all about what I didn't have. I didn't have drugs, I didn't have fun, I didn't have purpose, passion, excitement or adventure. You really don't want this kind

> My biggest fear while on drugs was to end up living a boring nine-to-five existence, to not be free. But, for some bizarre reason that is exactly the life I set up for myself. I pretended to be straight. I turned into my own worst nightmare.

My life after drugs was all about what I didn't have. I didn't have drugs, I didn't have fun, I didn't have purpose, passion, excitement or adventure. You really don't want this kind of environment, because drugs become the magic solution that can change all of that within seconds.

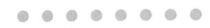

of environment, because drugs become the magic solution that can change all of that within seconds.

One Friday evening I came home from another long, disheartening day of youth work to find an old friend visiting. With her was a biker who had just got out of jail. I instantly liked him. He looked like an outlaw, with massive silver rings, a headband, leather vest, tattoos and a brash, outgoing personality. He unapologetically ate red meat, smoked like a chimney and swore like a trooper. He was true to himself and didn't give a damn what people thought.

I had been going through one of my periods of trying to be 'pure'. In my mind I had given up drugs and it had been months since I'd had alcohol. He instantly reminded me of everything I was missing out on. He offered me a beer and I decided to have one. It tasted incredible. I could feel my life force coming back so I had another. A few drinks later I decided to stuff being pure and had a cigarette. It felt good, really good. By the sixth beer tiredness hit. I was out of practice and was going to have to go to bed. Then he put out a line of speed for himself and his girlfriend. He asked me if I wanted some. I did, more than anything. I decided I would just have a taste though, half a line, then I'd get up early the next day and swim off any negative after-effects.

He put a line out for me to snort and it was sensational. I felt immortal. I was pulsating with euphoria, excitement and energy. Everything I had been missing was back. I was complete. This was what life was supposed to be like. I did another line and we decided to go to the pub. As soon as we got there I scored a bag of speed for myself, then two more, then we drank and snorted speed nonstop for the next two days. Reality didn't hit until I got back home on Sunday afternoon. Shock, depression and fear smothered me. I couldn't believe I had done it again. All the effort to be good had been wasted. I felt so worthless I thought about killing myself.

Instead I forced myself to go to bed, but there was too much speed in my system and I couldn't sleep. The next morning I couldn't get up to exercise. My head was spinning, and I was dizzy and nauseous. Despite serious paranoia and a mouth so dry I could barely speak, I made myself go to work. Somehow I fumbled through the day, terrified that at any moment I'd be exposed and fired. Every speed relapse I had I thought would be the last, but that one really was. I never did it again. It just wasn't worth the hangovers. My hard-drug-taking ended in an unresolved mix of sickness and confusion.

CONSTANT CRAVINGS

I quit speed because I wanted to give up the bad feelings, not because I wanted to give up the great feelings. This applies to every drug-taker. Because you are not supposed to have enjoyed drugs, replacing pleasure and excitement and euphoria does not factor in recovery programs. It never crossed my mind that I could get the great feelings back without drugs. The upshot was an insatiable hunger for those good feelings. Cravings became my new companion. I craved the memory of the good speed trips, the fullness and richness of those experiences.

> I quit speed because I wanted to give up the bad feelings, not because I wanted to give up the great feelings.

But it was more than that. I missed the whole thing—the ceremony, the process of mixing it up in the spoon, the cigarette filter, the lighter, the look of it in the needle, flicking the air bubbles, the anticipation. It was like foreplay, then the sharp prick of the needle and slowly entering the vein knowing that in the next minute I would be in paradise, a climax beyond any orgasm. Absence led to heartache. Speed had its own presence, its own life. It was always there for me. It followed me everywhere, whispering promises of instant perfection, instant fulfilment.

Alexander Shulgin, who created many new psychoactive compounds, talked about how, in the process of manufacture, each compound would take on a personality, a real character of its own. He said it could be described as an 'entity' that could have either a dark or friendly nature.[1] I had that connection with speed. When I quit, I might have left the drug but it didn't leave me. It turned into a stalker drug. I constantly thought about taking it, but as soon as I recalled the horrendous hangovers, my immediate reaction was 'no'. This would be instantly followed by the alluring thought that maybe it would be good and magic, like it used to be, and I would think about taking it again. This dialogue circled endlessly in my head. I had no control over it. It drove me mad.

THE LOVE/DRUG CONNECTION

In traditional Chinese philosophy, the basic elements of the material world are wood, fire, earth, metal and water. Each organ is associated with an element. The heart, for example, belongs to the fire element. Drugs force the fire to burn brightly, which is why you can take ecstasy, cocaine or speed and feel overwhelming love, inspiration and excitement. This is also one of the reasons why you feel you have a *relationship* with a drug.

However, these drugs overstimulate and harm the heart and fire element. Depression, anxiety, insomnia and emptiness are the result, and this is one of the reasons why you feel grief after you give up. You can take more drugs to try and make the pain go away, but eventually it cannot be corrected artificially by substances. The only option is to *heal* the organs. The heart is the seat of love. Unless you heal the heart you won't feel love again or be able to love yourself or anyone else.

Drugs are all about feelings. Like most drug users I lived in the world of the emotions. Everything I did was based on how I felt. When I was on drugs I was happy when I was high. When I finally gave up drugs everyone else was happy because I was clean, but I felt terrible. This wasn't only due to organ damage. My life on drugs was mapped out. I was constantly calculating when I could do my next drug or alcohol binge, how long it would take to recover, how good I would feel and so on. After quitting, all of that was gone. There was no direction in my life. I went to work every day and went through the motions, but felt like I didn't know what I was doing anymore.

Another problem in my life after drugs was that I had been gone from the straight world for the better part of a decade. The normal development and plan-making phase of people my age had passed me by. Families and careers had not been of interest to me. People told me I was immature, but that stuff simply doesn't matter when you are high. Once the drugs were gone, the present was too painful and I didn't have any concept of a future. It was a big empty space, so I had to take up drinking again to try and fill it up.

One of my work colleagues, a recovering alcoholic, convinced me to go to a meeting with him so I could speak openly about how I felt to like-minded people to lift my spirits. As soon as we arrived I regretted it. A group of grim-looking people were sitting around on plastic chairs chain-smoking. They all appeared resigned and defeated. There was no spirit there, no inspiration. My first thought was that I didn't want to be like that. I didn't want to live a soul-destroying half-life.

Most importantly, I didn't want to admit to my family that I was an alcoholic and addict, and that I had done something wrong. They might not have been drug users or binge drinkers, but they were the standard dysfunctional post-war European family riddled with questionable behaviours. It seemed hypocritical that they didn't have to admit to wrongdoing but I did, just because I took drugs. I left the meeting feeling angry but also confused. I knew it was a system that helped thousands and thousands of people, but I couldn't connect with it on any level.

BACK TO NORMAL

I didn't want to take speed or other drugs, but I still wanted to drink if I felt like it. I didn't want to be a recovered addict, I just wanted to be normal again—having dinner with people without having to get blind drunk first, meeting friends on the weekend for barbecues and being happy to drink mineral water or a couple of light beers, and perhaps an occasional joint just for a laugh. I wanted to feel fulfilled and at peace, rather than tortured and needing to numb myself.

Being normal also meant having real friends, not just people to take drugs or drink with. For years I had been socialising with people whose lives were as messed up as mine. Their homes looked like mine and, like me, they had no plans. Many were ex-hippies who had become alcoholics. Our grounds for interaction were being drunk or stoned, and when I stopped smoking and drinking I couldn't be around them anymore, because we no longer had anything in common.

I made new friends who had structured lives and plans. They invited me to join in on fishing trips, sporting events, go-kart racing and parties. I would make a huge effort to enjoy myself, but try as I might, I could only sustain interest and a positive attitude for about fifteen minutes before everything became bland and uninspiring again. I knew if I had some speed I would have been able to get into anything. Without drugs I felt totally disengaged from life.

My goal was to look as if I was having a good time but it was false, so it was exhausting. I couldn't be my real self, because my real self was depressed and in pain. I didn't like shopping centres, clubs or barbecues. My real self had no passion for life, other than being stoned or drunk. Non-drug users don't understand so I couldn't tell any of my new friends how I really felt. Drug users or drinkers would have understood, but I couldn't talk to them because I wasn't doing drugs or binge drinking anymore.

At that time in my life, I came to the conclusion that my drug-taking must have ruined me. Drugs had made me aware of the multi-dimensional nature of life in our universe. They showed me how rich and beautiful life could be. They had allowed me access into dimensions and realities far beyond the physical. I had seen worlds non-drug users could never imagine. Drugs revealed the enormous abundance of the universe. High on speed or LSD everything was possible, everything was about unlimited expansion. For me that was the real world. It was my current life that was false. Drugs had been the best part of my life. Life after drugs was a major disappointment on every level. It made me think I had been better off on drugs.

THE RAINBOW BRIDGE

Then I found my solution. A notice in the local newspaper advertised a talk the following Sunday by a spiritual teacher who was coming to town. I looked forward to it all week. When I finally got there it was a bit different to what I had imagined. The venue was a room in the local pub, and an aroma of beer and cigarettes filled the air. There were about forty people in the room from a variety of backgrounds. The teacher asked us to prepare ourselves by closing our eyes and listening to the music. He pushed a button and panpipe music filled the room. The tape occasionally slowed down distorting the sound but I tried not to let it distract me. As my mind started to drift, I was jolted back to reality by someone vigorously shaking my hand. I jumped in surprise and opened my eyes. The teacher was right in front of me, his face inches from mine. Up close he had crazy lobster eyes which seemed to go in different directions.

Despite the strangeness of it all there was something about him that appealed to me. He explained he was travelling the countryside introducing people to the technique referred to as the rainbow bridge, which allowed you access to higher worlds of liberation, joy and abundance. Just what I needed, a bridge out of my misery to a world of light and energy. He said the process would open up the third eye. It would take seven weeks to develop the bridge, one for each chakra, so we all had to come every Sunday for the next two months. After that, our lives would never be the same. This suited me perfectly. I didn't want one more day of my life as it was.

He initiated us that day. We were supposed to close our eyes during this process, but I squinted through my eyelids to see what he was doing. He was standing at the front of the room, his arms outstretched and his lips moving. He was swaying backwards and forwards. To my surprise I could feel a faint warmth moving through me, which slowly grew and was very pleasurable. This was my first experience of what I thought was a sacred force without the use of psychedelic drugs. For the rest of that day I felt very clear and emotionally supported—even my family commented on how different I seemed. I was thrilled. This was exactly what I needed in my life.

The next week I made sure I got there early so I could sit in the front row, as the room had been full the week before. This time only five people turned up. Everything was the same, except the tape was a bit more chewed-up. The teacher said we all had to become vegetarians and stop drinking alcohol. This was fantastic. Now I would be forced never to drink again and could really become spiritual. He then added there was to be no sex of any sort. I was the only male in the group and he looked at me meaningfully as he said this. I assumed he meant no masturbation either, so I decided I would be really pure and give this up too.

After four weeks there were only three of us left. By then I was starting to feel light-headed and confused and I kept experiencing dizzy spells. It was like a permanent, low-level speed hangover. I told myself that it was part of the purification, that it must have been my bad past coming out. Plus, I was addicted to the great energy transmission each session started with.

The next week my symptoms became worse. The teacher said to stick with it. On the way home that day I stopped at a supermarket. When I burst into tears in the frozen goods aisle, for no apparent reason, I knew I couldn't do it anymore. The spiritual path was not for me after all. I felt hopeless, but also secretly relieved as I could now go back to a limited way of living that I was more comfortable with.

> The spiritual path was not for me after all. I felt hopeless, but also secretly relieved as I could now go back to a limited way of living that I was more comfortable with.

My failure at spirituality drove me to drink heavily again, but in a weird way that is what put me back on track. The following week I spotted an exotic-looking woman sitting at the bar by herself. In my mind she evoked images of spirituality and mysticism. Despite my self-doubt I went over to talk to her. We were immediately engaged in a deep and meaningful discussion. Around Sonia I sensed purpose, destiny and completion. When the pub closed that night she came home with me.

Late the next morning I staggered out of bed to find her and my car gone. She reappeared later saying she had been to see her grandmother on some important spiritual business. This happened a few more times over the next couple of days. Being with her made me feel positive and uplifted, so I invited her to a family barbecue. She turned up with her boyfriend. I felt devastated and used. She hadn't been visiting her grandmother each time she left me— she had been with her boyfriend.

Later on one of my relatives struck up a conversation with Sonia's boyfriend and they hit it off. He dumped Sonia and left with my relative. I felt as if I was trapped in some sort of terrible soap opera. When my relative returned the next day, she had a brochure for a college of natural medicine that the ex-boyfriend of my ex-girlfriend had given her. As she handed it to me I felt a surge of energy rush through me. I had a moment of absolute clarity and knew the brochure was somehow connected with my destiny.

14 DOWN AND OUT

Going to college and studying would give my life purpose. I eagerly gathered the information about courses offered, then made myself enrol in acupuncture. I was very nervous as I had tried to enrol in a university course before but hadn't gone through with it because when I walked through the campus, filled with crowds of happy, intelligent people who really seemed to have their lives together, I knew I didn't belong there. My paranoia and low self-esteem meant that being with anyone who was engaged in and passionate about life was hugely stressful for me. I was only ever relaxed in the company of real down-and-outers—society's outcasts. In that university environment I would have felt judged and watched the whole time. I couldn't do it.

A college of natural medicine would be a bigger challenge. There would be thousands of happy, intelligent and *pure* people all in one spot. I was sure none of them would have done drugs or stuffed up their lives. But this time I couldn't give in to the fear because I was running out of good reasons to keep living and something had to change. This time the pain of not doing it would be worse than the

> My paranoia and low self-esteem meant that being with anyone who was engaged in and passionate about life was hugely stressful for me. I was only ever relaxed in the company of real down-and-outers–society's outcasts.

pain of doing it, so I forced myself to go through the enrolment process and immediately ordered all the course textbooks, thinking that this would make me follow through. Classes didn't start for several months, so my plan was to work two jobs and spend that time getting really fit and healthy. I wanted to turn up at college in good shape, work really hard, get through the course and become a top graduate. If I could do that I was sure my life would be great and I would, at last, be accepted by others. Most importantly, my family would see I was a worthwhile person.

Getting fit and healthy meant giving up the binge drinking. That was tough. Alcohol had become almost more necessary than food for me. My body screamed for the taste of it. I couldn't sleep. My hands shook constantly, my face twitched. I was scattered, stirred up, edgy and unsettled. I had to make huge detours through town so that I never passed the pub. Just the sight of it made me feel grief. I exercised obsessively to keep the cravings at bay.

LIVING IN FEAR

On my first day of college I arrived an hour early for my nine thirty lecture. I stood at the front gate trying to get the nerve to walk in. I hadn't slept for two nights because I was so worried about being around pure people. I felt like vomiting. I forced myself in, then stumbled to the reception area. I was shaking so much I had to hang on to the counter. Finally, I managed to ask what room my lecture was in.

I had to go through a large cafeteria to get there. I was sure everyone was staring at me. I felt so naked, so fucked-up. I knew I didn't belong there. How in hell was I supposed to help other people? It was a joke.

Then I found the lecture room and it was full. I sat outside to gather my courage. An older man came over and started chatting to me, casually asking me how I was going and what I was doing. Suddenly I realised that he was the lecturer and panic washed over me. I tried to answer his questions but tripped on my words. Then he said, 'Come on, let's go in.' To my absolute horror I had to walk in with him, in front of everyone. My knees were like jelly and

I had a desperate urge to urinate. I made it to the back of the room and sat down in the furthest corner, still trembling. I thought I would have to force myself to sit through the lecture, but within minutes I was captivated. The lecturer talked about divination, alchemy, ghosts, emperors, martial artists and the art of healing. He presented a picture of a world without limitation where every possibility could manifest. It was a world in which you could change your destiny by cultivating your life force. This was like drug talk. It engaged my heart, body and soul. I knew that if I followed this through I would find my way forward in life.

> The lecturer talked about divination, alchemy, ghosts, emperors, martial artists and the art of healing. He presented a picture of a world without limitation where every possibility could manifest. It was a world in which you could change your destiny by cultivating your life force. This was like drug talk.

I remember looking at the lecturer and thinking that my greatest dream would be to be so together, so normal that I could stand in front of a crowd of people and speak passionately about a topic in which I was expert. Years later, after becoming a lecturer myself, I found out the lecturer that day was very nervous, and was pleased to have found me outside the seminar room. He was experiencing normal fear or nerves. I had 'ex-drug user fear', an uncontrollable and irrational fear rising out of my depleted kidneys and organs. It ran riot through me and went on for years. It was one of the worst post-drug symptoms. Because I was more introverted at the time, or yin, I experienced high levels of timidity that I constantly had to push through. Yang types respond to the fear with aggressive behaviour.

PARTY PERSON

After getting through that first day, I knuckled down and became totally focused on my goal of becoming a successful acupuncturist. While working day and night on my studies, I consoled myself with the idea that one day I would give myself a 'reward'. I'd have a big party night where I would really let go, get drunk and behave foolishly. I'd be in the moment and part of everything again. Drugs and alcohol were what made you feel good in life. My reward would be to have them again. But it wasn't until my third year of college that I got around to doing it.

I carefully planned the whole evening: the venue, what drinks I would have and even the taxi ride home. I invited a group of people and off we went. We all ordered drinks, but my first beer after three years made me feel uneasy. Deciding I was out of practice I ordered a few more to warm me up, but each beer made me feel worse. By the time I got to the fifth I thought I was going to faint. I tried smoking a cigarette, but that made me nauseous. After about an hour I had to go home. My vision of being able to set my real self free collapsed. Worse still, people thought I was weird, again, because I couldn't drink and have fun like a normal person.

HEALING ADDICTION

The next morning I was utterly disillusioned. Throughout all the years of emptiness and confusion I knew I could always use drugs and alcohol to make me feel fulfilled. It was my safety net. Now I was a substance abuser for whom substances no longer worked.

Thinking about it I realised I was living in a very different way to what most people would after drug or alcohol addiction. I was actively building physical, emotional and spiritual health. As an acupuncturist you are supposed to exemplify the health and high energy you want your patients to have, and thus inspire them to be like you. Because of my self-esteem and fear issues, I was highly motivated to do this, so I built my chi daily. I ate only healthy food, I did tai-chi, deep breathing and exercised. I took powerful supplements daily and Chinese raw herbs each week and, because as students we frequently practised on each other, I was having therapeutic massage or acupuncture several times a week. Because of this my organs had been slowly rebuilding. My system had become more refined and was now rejecting alcohol and cigarettes of its

Because of the steps I took to exemplify health and high energy, my organs had been slowly rebuilding. My system had become more refined and was now rejecting alcohol and cigarettes of its own volition. I wanted to drink and party but my body didn't want me to. Without knowing it, I had been doing exactly what was needed to start healing addiction. I was an addict who was no longer attracted to alcohol or drugs. If everyone was wrong about me being an addict for life, what else were they wrong about?

own volition. I wanted to drink and party but my body didn't want me to. Without knowing it, I had been doing exactly what was needed to start healing addiction. I was an addict who was no longer attracted to alcohol or drugs. If everyone was wrong about me being an addict for life, what else were they wrong about?

● ● ● ● ● ● ● ●

15 NO MAN'S LAND

All through college, even though I studied from morning until night, I felt empty. Once I graduated and set up my acupuncture clinic, I knew all of that would change. And it did, but only while I was working on clients. Between patient sessions I was lost again. The job, business and friends were not enough—something was missing. I kept thinking that things would change, that tomorrow would be a better day, but tomorrow would come and it would be the same all over again. Nothing ever changed. I felt like I was a ghost, but wasn't dead yet. I sensed there was another option but the door was always locked. Finally, I discovered that acknowledging my loneliness and pain was the key to open that door.

> I felt like I was a ghost, but wasn't dead yet. I sensed there was another option but the door was always locked. Finally, I discovered that acknowledging my loneliness and pain was the key to open that door.

Processing my stored pain was the way out. But I didn't know how. I had been to counsellors and tried various new age therapies but nothing seemed to make any difference. Then I accidentally discovered the way out. A friend was supposed to meet me at the movies one night, but she couldn't make it so I ended up going alone. It was one of those devastating French tragedies all about heartbreak, isolation and rejection. It really delved deep into fundamental human pain. As I sat there absorbed in the agony of the characters in the film, I was able to sink into my own pain. Out in the external world, I felt I was supposed to be happy and normal. The film put me into a zone where I could acknowledge these feelings in myself. Instead of frantically trying to suppress them, I let them surface. When I did that, I felt so real that getting to know my pain became my new passion.

Winston Churchill, who used to suffer depression, famously referred to bouts of it as visits from the black dog. Rather than sitting there and letting the dog run the show, I decided to take charge. Just as in my drug-taking days when I'd go out on my highs, I started to take my lows out. I would deliberately spend my days off by myself. If there were no suitable movies I would drive somewhere isolated and just sit and let my pain come forward until it consumed me. Then I would transcend it, and let the next wave come forward. I really let myself feel my isolation and hopelessness. Finally I started to feel at home with pain.

> I would deliberately spend my days off by myself. If there were no suitable movies I would drive somewhere isolated and just sit and let my pain come forward until it consumed me.

> You need to be able to accept your post-drug lows without resisting them, just as you used to accept your drug highs.

● ● ● ● ● ● ● ●

THE ART OF PROCESSING PAIN

You need to be able to accept your post-drug lows without resisting them, just as you used to accept your drug highs. This is not an easy process as, generally speaking, we fear pain, which we have been conditioned to suppress with medication. For drug users there is the additional complication that post-drug pain is invisible, uncharted and misunderstood. If you break a leg or have an operation people expect you to recover over a certain period of time. But drug use generates far more subtle and complex symptoms, ranging from delusion to simple exhaustion. Speed might make you feel temporarily terrific, energetic and lively, but it draws upon your own energy stores to do this. A night on speed could use up the energy needed over an entire week of normal life. The more often you take drugs, the further you tax your inner resources that will have to be replaced one day.

For drug users there is the additional complication that post-drug pain is invisible, uncharted and misunderstood.

After drugs, some people just want to sit there, not get out of bed, not move, and not talk to anyone for very, very long periods of time. The body calls on these states to provide an opportunity to retreat and heal. Non-drug users have no idea what ex-addicts are going through. Partners, parents and friends often react inappropriately. During the period when I spent my days off watching French tragedies or wandering around parks with my headphones on getting into feeling lonely, people told me my behaviour was not healthy, that I was becoming a hermit. One of my relatives even had the nerve to tell me that I used to be much more fun when I was on drugs.

Non-drug users have no idea what ex-addicts are going through.

Pain is a natural part of life and it is important to understand it and take away the fear of feeling it. Feeling it is part of it, but you also need to be in a situation where you can transform it. When I work on patients, I use acupuncture points and chi flow to put them into an altered or dream-like state, so they can face their pain without resistance. Doing chi-gung, tai-chi and meditation every day taught me to alter my own state naturally, so that I could face my pain without getting caught in it. Instead, I could acknowledge and free it.

The only reason I was able to successfully process my pain by myself was because I had this training in place. I would not recommend processing pain to anyone unless they have the necessary skills. If you face too much emotional pain on your own, without transformational techniques or a therapist to guide you through, you can get trapped in it.

LIFE IN LIMBO

Once I started acknowledging and releasing my pain, things became clearer. After drugs and alcohol I had ended up in no man's land, a limbo. My whole focus had been on getting back to normality, or life as it was before drugs. I had missed the most important point. Limbo is a *transition* place between worlds in which the old has died but the new has not been born yet. From limbo you don't go backwards. You move forwards to a new place.

Once this sank in, it registered that limbo, or no man's land, can be the stepping stone to a world so spectacular and miraculous that it is hard to comprehend. *Everyone* can go there, regardless of where they have been or what they have done. Processing your pain is your ticket to this new place. The whole point of us being here is to grow. Pain encourages us to change so it is an opportunity for growth. Our physical body is the means by which we do this.

> The whole point of us being here is to grow. Pain encourages us to change so it is an opportunity for growth. Our physical body is the means by which we do this.

NAVIGATING NO MAN'S LAND

Every ex-drug user is going to have to cross no man's land. Given my time again, I would tackle this as if I was an explorer about to go on a great expedition. Rather than stumbling dazed through a decade of cravings, alcohol, pills and suicidal depression, I would organise maps, equipment and supplies. I would acknowledge and accept my past, and find the value in it, rather than pretending it didn't happen or getting stuck trying to work out where I went wrong. That is not the right frame of mind in which to start any journey, let alone the post-drug journey.

I'd accept the hardships because the thrill of heading to a magical place, and the insights along the way, was going to make it all worthwhile. I would also look for 'post-drug peers', people who have given up drugs, crossed no man's land, then recaptured what they wanted in life without drugs. You need people who can inspire you to keep going. The better prepared you are for your life after drugs, the more chance you have of staying off drugs permanently.

If you have been a heavy drug user, you can't just sit around after you quit and hope to go back to normal because, for most people, it won't happen. Once you have started buying highs with good quality drugs, you have to keep going down that path. You have to be prepared to buy post-drug highs by actively investing in your health every day. But the new highs are going to be worth every cent.

> The better prepared you are for your life after drugs, the more chance you have of staying off drugs permanently.

PART IV:
HOW TO LIVE AFTER DRUGS

16 POST-DRUG HIGHS AND LOWS

The one person who should understand the cycle of highs and lows is an ex-drug user. If you do a weekend on ecstasy or speed or ice, you are not surprised to feel bad mid-week—it's part of the package. You know it is not permanent and that by Friday you will feel good again. You don't resist it. When you feel bad you don't go out and then spend the evening sitting there agonising over the fact. You know you need a few quiet days. You stay at home. You watch TV and smoke and drink. When you are on drugs you accept and understand the lows. This same strategy needs to be applied to the lows after quitting drugs, because even if you rest, eat well, take supplements, have regular therapeutic treatment and do all the right things, hard days will still happen.

> When you are on drugs you accept and understand the lows. This same strategy needs to be applied to the lows after quitting drugs, because even if you rest, eat well, take supplements, have regular therapeutic treatment and do all the right things, hard days will still happen.

POST-DRUG DEPRESSION

Shane was twenty-eight. He managed a busy restaurant and worked long hours each day. He had been a speed user for a few years, but had been off drugs for a couple of months. He had been doing all the right things to buy back the highs: the regular therapeutic massage, the powerful supplements and exercising each morning. Everything seemed manageable but then he hit a 'bad' day. It was a Sunday, his day off. He woke up depressed, tired and frustrated. His body ached and he had no interest in getting out of bed, let alone exercising or taking supplements. He forced himself to get up and tried to snap himself out of it, but everything made him feel like crying.

Shane had been invited to a friend's place that afternoon for a small party and felt obligated to go. He tried to be sociable, but after half an hour he couldn't maintain the front, so he went back home. He wandered around the house, then sat chain-smoking, drinking coffee and staring at the TV. Nothing changed so he took a sleeping pill and went to bed, hoping to wake up in a better emotional place.

Shane thought he must have done something wrong to feel so bad. Everything had been going so well and all of a sudden he'd hit a wall. What he didn't know was, these feelings are a natural part of the post-drug healing process. When you have a day off, the body knows it and sees an opportunity to retreat and to heal some of the damage done by drugs. Some suppressed pain surfaces as part of this. Shane thought he shouldn't indulge in the pain and should get on with life. But, as I explained to him, that Sunday his body had released a manageable amount of pain to be processed. When this happens, don't force yourself to go out, socialise and expend energy if you don't feel like it. Try to be comfortable with your discomfort, because this is what processes the pain.

THE ZIGZAG PATH

Shane had been working really hard on his recovery. He was experiencing constant improvement and thought if he kept all his treatment up this would continue. When he hit that bad day he thought he had 'lost it all'. But traditional Chinese medicine shows us health and improvement is always three steps forward and one back. The post-drug high graph is the reverse of the drug high graph. The post-drug high graph starts at the base line of depression then inclines, falls then inclines again. Each peak is higher than the subsequent fall. If you draw a line connecting the peaks and the lows, you have a big fat line that constantly ascends. The great news is that it can keep going right off the chart upwards into infinity.

I suggested to Shane that on the days he felt bad, he try and sit with his emotions and avoid distractions that overrode his feelings. Instead he might want to read books about triumph over adversity—in particular books where the authors use practices such as chi-gung or yoga to transform painful lives into bliss and happiness. If he wanted to watch TV, rather than mindless entertainment he could perhaps choose a film about a boxer who beat the odds, or people who achieve great things in the face of obstacles.

The post-drug high graph starts at the base line of depression then inclines, falls then inclines again. Each peak is higher than the subsequent fall. If you draw a line connecting the peaks and the lows, you have a big fat line that constantly ascends. The great news is that it can keep going right off the chart upwards into infinity.

CIGARETTES AND GRIEF

I also recommended that Shane try to cut down on cigarettes and coffee on those days. In traditional Chinese medicine cigarettes are connected with the metal element and the lungs and colon. The lungs are responsible for accepting the past, living in the now and embracing the future. The colon is associated with 'letting go', which is why some people need cigarettes to have a bowel movement. Emotionally, the lungs are also associated with sadness and grief. When you give up a drug or alcohol habit you will naturally face grief, sadness and loss.

Because cigarettes engage the lungs they can create a feeling of acceptance of

When you give up a drug or alcohol habit you will naturally face grief, sadness and loss.

the moment and appear to ease emotional distress. Ex-addicts often chain-smoke for this reason. I also see non-drug users who finally quit smoking cigarettes, then find they cannot stop crying afterwards. Cigarettes might fill an emotional hole, but they also stop you processing the pain. When I quit drugs I smoked heavily and drank coffee by the gallon. Coffee is a stimulant, so it picks up your energy and it also temporarily takes away that sense of pain and emptiness. At times when you want to retreat within and process, I would reduce both. It is not about giving up coffee and cigarettes, it is about reducing your intake on that day to get a bit more familiar with your discomfort.

Ex-addicts often chain-smoke for this reason.
I also see non-drug users who finally quit smoking cigarettes, then find they cannot stop crying afterwards.

After drugs, the cycle of highs and lows will continue, but this time the highs will come out of working with the lows.

I suggested that on his post-drug low days Shane use the same tactics that he used on his drug-taking low days. He didn't have to actively get into his depression or sadness, nor did he have to go out and try to have a good time. The trick is to *respect* how you feel and know it will pass. After drugs, the cycle of highs and lows will continue, but this time the highs will come out of working with the lows.

17 ENGAGING WITH CRAVINGS

A major issue after drugs is cravings. It has been estimated that of people who get off drugs through recovery programs, at least eighty percent go back to drugs within a year. Cravings are seen as a primary cause, and suppressing cravings is seen as a key part of recovery. However, after treating quite a few clients who had issues with cravings it became apparent how they can be harnessed as part of the healing process. I came to realise that cravings are a powerful motivating force that can help you achieve your post-drug high.

Paul, who had been a heroin addict for years, got me thinking along these lines. He'd finally given up and was sure he was on top of everything. He had no plan to deal with his cravings, though. When they hit, all he could think about was heroin. He decided he wasn't ready to stop. I asked Paul if he could imagine getting into the heroin mind-set again, of devoting all his time to finding money, scoring and using heroin every day, of living with a sole focus on getting high. I often use these scenarios with clients because it helps them clarify how they really feel. Paul reacted instantly with a negative. He definitely didn't want to live for heroin anymore.

> I came to realise that cravings are a powerful motivating force that can help you achieve your post-drug high.

A second therapeutic option is controlled drug use with a view to gradually stopping. This approach isn't for everyone. It only works if you are physically active and engaged, and not able to get drugs whenever you want them. Some people use occupations where drug-testing is in place to control their drug intake, or work in remote areas. It takes a lot of mental strength, though, because the weeks without the drug are really tough, especially the first few days of each 'off' period.

Paul said he couldn't imagine living that kind of life, of ongoing bingeing and withdrawing. When I asked about his current lifestyle, he said he had moved back to his parents' home. He had no job and his girlfriend had left him, so he had no reason to get up and nothing to do all day. He had been living for heroin, and now had a big blank space in his life where heroin had been. This is not a situation in which you will be able to control cravings, and if you do give in and use drugs again, it can ruin the high because you hate yourself for being so weak. It's a lose-lose deal.

In my opinion Paul really had finished with drugs. His passion for heroin was gone but he hadn't given his heart anything else to attach to, so his cravings were ruling him. Cravings are connected with the heart and spleen. The heart/ fire element is linked with spirit and purpose. To feel fulfilment you need to have the fire burning brightly. The spleen/earth provides the fuel to be burned. If the spleen doesn't have this fuel, which is partially derived from the food you eat, it reminds you something is missing—you feel hungry. Hard drugs are such a powerful source of fuel that your fire element burns so brightly you feel as if all your desires are met. At the same time it empties your fuel tanks. Knowing this, the spleen reminds you that something is missing, but this time the something it suggests is drugs, as this is what has been the basis of your fuel. Cravings are powerful spiritual, physiological and emotional urges that are focused purely on what you are missing. While they can be hard to fight against, they can also be a powerful force to harness.

WORKING WITH CRAVINGS

Like Paul, my relationship with drugs ended but my cravings didn't. Initially I couldn't handle them so I used drugs again. Later I controlled them by building my organ health and strength, and staying fully occupied and stimulated. At home I covered the walls of my room with diagrams of the meridian systems of traditional Chinese medicine, posters of tai-chi masters and anything else I could find that reinforced my vision of my future. But as soon as I was out of that environment or not working, the cravings returned.

Cravings are powerful spiritual, physiological and emotional urges that are focused purely on what you are missing. While they can be hard to fight against, they can also be a powerful force to harness.

Then came the magical day that the cravings vanished. I was driving home after a long day when I noticed I was in that great state where you feel all of your needs have been met. It was like a drug state. At first I thought I was just numb from overwork, but then realised I felt whole, complete. It was the most real 'whole' feeling I had ever felt, more whole than any drug made me feel. That was the day that Jules, my first drug client, came in. That was the day I began to accept my past and clearly understood my purpose. And that was the day I had some subconscious recognition that there is a spiritual aspect to cravings.

My discovery of traditional Chinese medicine and covering my walls with reminders of my path assisted the fire element to burn brightly. Along with the good food I was eating and the Chinese herbs, it fed my spleen with plenty of good material to digest into fuel for my heart. This temporarily countered physical cravings. That they went at exactly the same time I started working with drugs again and discovered my real purpose as a therapist was no accident. As I explained to Paul, cravings have a physical as well as a spiritual aspect. You can treat the physical with spleen-building herbs, supplements, medicinal diet and acupuncture. Then to treat the emotional or spiritual aspect, you need to understand and pursue your soul purpose, so that your fire element can burn brightly again.

HEALING THE HEART

Inspiration is a major factor in post-drug healing. It is an emotion belonging to the heart. Being inspired helps redress the weaknesses or imbalances in the heart and the fire element. So if Paul wanted to stay off heroin, he had to make major changes in his lifestyle. He would have to structure his day, build his life energy but also identify and then pursue the things that inspired him.

When I asked about this he said he had always wanted to study audio engineering and composing, but had never followed up on this. Heroin had taken away the last shreds of his self-worth so he didn't think he deserved this future. But the heroin had also finished off a chapter of his life and it was time to embark on a new path and build a new future, by following up on that dream. Now Paul had no choice. Heroin addiction had taken him to rock bottom. He had to recreate himself in accord with his true desires. If you stop drugs, then don't do anything, it is easy to feel you have wasted your life.

Music is a great strategy to heal the heart. In eastern spiritual traditions monks often play instruments to activate the heart. They may be in a loving relationship with the divine but that is an abstract relationship; playing an instrument is the physical application, and it strengthens the heart. Inspiration and excitement can be generated by any form of creative activity. Many clients say that they are not creative, but we are all creative and we all have rhythm—it is an integral part of human nature. I am not suggesting taking up a hobby here. You have to make creative practice an essential part of life after drugs.

This all sounds good in theory but the hardest thing is to start. If you are an ex-user, once you identify what inspires you, act on that impulse without thinking about it, otherwise fear and doubt will overshadow you. Never look back. Go and enrol in a course. If a full-time commitment is not possible start with a weekend, evening or casual class. It doesn't matter what it is so long as you commit to it, then turn up. As soon as you get there it will feel good. When you choose growth the universe will support your actions, but you have to make the first move. Surrounding yourself with as much visual support as possible will make it easier. Plaster your walls with pictures of the lifestyle you desire. Avoid people who resist and oppose your intent to change until you are strong enough to withstand the pressure.

METHADONE AND CRAVINGS

Sarah had been a long-term heroin user who wanted to give up heroin but was too scared to go cold turkey, so she sought medical help and had been prescribed methadone to avoid the heroin withdrawal and cravings. It was supposed to ease her off heroin but she ended up being on methadone for six years. Now she wanted to get off that but was really scared of the withdrawal, which she said was going to be even worse than a heroin withdrawal.

Methadone is a synthetic opiate. It does not produce the euphoria of heroin, but it does counter cravings, which is the most common cause of relapse. Treating heroin addiction with another, even more addictive drug is not a long-term solution. On methadone Sarah might not be craving heroin, but she lacked motivation, had severe memory loss, bad teeth, experienced massive weight gain and could not sleep.

Pulse and tongue diagnostics revealed that Sarah was blood deficient, kidney yang deficient and spleen deficient, which explained all her symptoms. These deficiencies, which I have seen in other long-term methadone users, can be treated with regular acupuncture, Chinese herbs prescribed by a good therapist and nutritional supplements. This is really important in the recovery process. Long-term drug users are seriously nutrient deprived but often have no desire for food. Herbs and supplements are like taking concentrated liquid food. They help build up the organs and reduce the severity of withdrawal symptoms.

Sarah felt as if her life was on hold, and in a way it was. The purpose of methadone is to suppress cravings, but when you engage with cravings positively, they can drive you forward to find purpose and meaning after drugs. There is no motivation more powerful than a drug craving. It makes you creative and it makes you find a way to get drugs. Addicts always achieve their goals and it is cravings that drive them to do this.

Each morning I used to wake with the singular goal of finding and using drugs and each day I achieved that. I had no doubt about my ability. During the period I was heavily dependent on alcohol, I woke up one morning on a yacht out at sea. I panicked momentarily, thinking I had been kidnapped by white-slavers before remembering that I'd volunteered to crew in a drunken binge the night before. A week later the boat docked thousands of kilometres from home. I had no money but was totally focused on getting enough alcohol each day to get by. It took me two weeks to hitchhike back home, but I managed to get drunk and stoned every day. Thanks to the cravings, I was a success strategist's dream.

My cravings had driven me relentlessly forward in my life on drugs, and in my life after drugs. They forced me to rebuild myself in line with my soul purpose and thus to finally feel fulfilled. Only then did they go. Without cravings I wouldn't have kept searching for my real purpose and would have resigned myself to a half-life. I now view cravings as the hunger pangs of the soul. Hunger draws your attention to something important you are missing. Cravings carry the message that your soul needs nourishment.

Hunger draws your attention to something important you are missing. Cravings carry the message that your soul needs nourishment.

18 HANDLING POST-DRUG VAGUENESS

When people give up drugs, they often feel vague and directionless, but ex-drug users cannot afford to feel like this. You need to know exactly where you stand at all times. While you are in rehab every moment is planned, so there is no room for vagueness. This is why people feel safe in that environment. They know exactly where they belong. They are fully occupied and their lives are structured.

After drugs you need to recreate that environment yourself. Inertia, vagueness and confusion will rule unless you take control. Find a settled environment. Drugs make you feel settled regardless of where you are. They provide a centre within the madness. After you give up, you need somewhere settled to replace that aspect of the drug's action. Make your environment as organised as possible. Get a good bed and sleep in the same place every night. If you settle the physical, the mind can follow more easily. Don't leave an empty day ahead of yourself. Get a plan, otherwise doubt, despair and defeat will take over along with cravings.

> Don't leave an empty day ahead of yourself. Get a plan, otherwise doubt, despair and defeat will take over along with cravings.

119

The most important thing to structure is the morning. The morning holds the secret to healing addiction. If you wake up and take charge between 5 am and 7 am, you can change your life. Each section of the day is ruled by an element that offers us different possibilities. Each morning between five and seven it is the time of the metal element, and it presents an opportunity for us to transform ourselves. Drugs initiate transformation. You can be instantly shifted from one state to another, or one reality to another. It is instantaneous, non-logical and non-linear movement. Drug users understand the concept of transformation, so you can make that knowledge work for you. By working with your inner transformative potential each morning, you can get back everything that the drugs gave you. In the old days you woke up for drugs, now you need to wake up for *yourself* and your purpose.

FINDING PURPOSE

When I finished with drugs I couldn't imagine doing what I am now. I just kept following up on anything that felt right. Step by step it led me to my destiny. All you need do is follow a glimpse or a seed of something, regardless of how inaccessible it might seem. It was an old brochure for a college of natural medicine that launched me onto my path. If you have no idea of your purpose, do something creative and constructive. Go to a bookshop or library and see what appeals. Look for something that will creatively engage you, such as tattooing, woodworking, photography, fashion or electronic music. Buy a book or magazine, follow your feelings and actively create something. By making things and problem-solving, you draw on your inner resources and spark inspiration.

Set yourself a goal and disregard all limiting thought patterns as they are a major post-drug problem. I constantly treat people who in their drug days were larger than life characters. They had wild hair, outfits and lifestyles. They ran huge rave parties or clubs and turned over tens of thousands of dollars a day. They really lived the abundance that drugs make you feel on every level. After drugs they would sit in front of me and tell me they couldn't do anything.

Something you wanted from drugs or felt on drugs will be linked to your life purpose. Get a whiteboard or notebook and write your ideas down until you work out what your purpose is. Most people won't know their purpose right away, so feel free to make changes whenever necessary. Keep the notebook with you or put the board somewhere where you see it all the time. This is a map for *you*. It is a physical reminder to refer to daily. The quicker you get a map the better, because in life after drugs happiness is not a default state. You need a plan to deliver happiness.

> Something you wanted from drugs or felt on drugs will be linked to your life purpose.

POST-DRUG PURPOSE

Chris had smoked dope for fifteen years. At first it made him feel free, but in the last few years marijuana started to generate panic and anxiety. He would get stoned, then become paranoid that he was about to have a heart attack. He started drinking vast amounts of alcohol before smoking, so that it wouldn't 'suffocate' him. Realising that something wasn't right with this picture, Chris gave up the dope. Since then he had been vague, directionless and confused.

Because he said marijuana had made him feel free, we looked at where he had encountered restraint in the past. Chris had dominating parents who were members of a cult religion. For Chris it was like being in an army camp. Everything was highly disciplined and rigid.

I have worked with quite a few people who have been in cults. The suppression of individual desires for the sake of group goals impacts on your ability to grow. Cults suppress the 'advance and act' qualities of the liver that are necessary to achieve your desires. Every time Chris tried to move towards something he wanted, the cult opposed it until he had no opinion about anything.

Chris hated this so he would leave the cult and smoke dope to be free again, only to feel he was doing something wrong. Overcome by guilt he would return to the cult and the cycle would start again. Finally he left for good, then got heavily into smoking dope. This was when the side-effects of panic and anxiety surfaced.

During the ten years Chris had been in the cult, marijuana allowed him to feel freedom, but it can only do that for a limited period of time. When that good feeling ran out, the magnifying quality of marijuana highlighted his underlying problem of suppression and restriction. His panic attacks and anxiety resulted from this and his underlying liver yang deficiency. He had been going through a constant cycle of repression and freedom. This had to be healed, and in his case that meant through personal development.

Chris was filling in time working casually as a handyman. His dream was to be a practitioner of natural medicine. He would get stoned and lie in bed, imagining life as a therapist. I asked what was stopping him, and he said lethargy, doubt and fear. He was worried he wouldn't get work, or wouldn't be able to make a living from it. Doubt and fear are normal when considering a new direction in life. In Chris' case it had become magnified due to his liver yang deficiency, which was also contributing to his inability to 'advance and act' to get his career underway. We needed to treat that through acupuncture, Chinese herbs and prescribed exercises.

Doubt and fear will continue to rise up in you even if you are on your path. When this happens to me I always ask, 'What is my alternative?' Chris knew what he wanted so being a casual handyman for the rest of his life was not going to make him happy. I said if he followed his dream he would have to have faith as well. Just because something is your purpose, it doesn't mean achieving it will be easy. Following your purpose can be extremely challenging, but the reward of pursuing it far outweighs the comfort of not trying.

Chris thought that studying natural medicine was his purpose, but it is not that simple. I thought becoming an acupuncturist was my purpose too, but you don't resolve issues simply by getting a new career. You don't resolve issues just by giving up drugs either. For Chris, resolution would come by identifying what organ imbalances he had and why. Then he could heal *himself,* regain assertiveness and true freedom, then apply the knowledge he gained from his own experiences and his studies to help others. This was his post-drug responsibility and purpose.

19 ECSTASY AND SPIRITUALITY

Spiritual practice is also an important part of life after drugs, as spirituality activates and heals the heart. But you need to be fit for the spiritual path. If you have had an extended period of heavy drug abuse you are probably not fit. My rainbow bridge experience demonstrated that for me. The damage the drugs did to my organs had not repaired and I was still drinking, smoking and eating badly. I didn't have the strength to handle an intense spiritual practice. Paradoxically, giving up smoking, drinking, meat and sex all at once put my system under further stress and made things even worse.

As many drug users have had intense spiritual experiences on drugs and do need to find that again in life after drugs, I suggest beginning by building organ strength and taking up a practice such as yoga or chi-gung. These take you on the path of spirituality by working with and strengthening the physical body. There are plenty of special forms of meditation around which can give you a high like a drug, but your organs need to be strong enough to process these experiences.

Malcolm, a wealthy and successful forty-year-old lawyer, was good-looking and athletic, with a mansion, a garage full of luxury cars, and adventure toys from speedboats to mountain bikes. He was a high-achiever, at the top of his class and profession, who had always lived for the future. At university he tried marijuana but it did nothing for him so he never took drugs again. Then when he went to London for a legal conference, he was offered ecstasy in a club some of the delegates had gone to. His immediate reaction was to say no, but for some reason he thought, why the hell not? Overwhelmed by love and joy, and feeling totally free, he danced unselfconsciously all night and bonded with everyone. It was the most extraordinary experience of his life. Malcolm had done extreme sports but the ecstasy experience was in a different league.

He was captivated and wanted more. He started using every weekend, graduating from one tablet a night to three-day bingeing sessions, followed by four days of recovery. He couldn't get enough, but the side-effects were getting more uncomfortable. He started taking time off work to recover. When he was at work his clients really annoyed him. His wife, a partner in the legal firm, was worried about him and the business, and told him to stop. Malcolm knew he was on a downward spiral, and had already toyed with trying ice and other drugs, so he forced himself to quit.

By the time Malcolm came to see me it was six months since his last ecstasy pill and he was miserable. He hated his job, his clients, his relationship and everything about his life. He only became a lawyer because his father, a successful lawyer himself, expected Malcolm to. Desperately missing the ecstasy highs, he tried extreme sports again, but nothing provided what the ecstasy had.

When I asked what he wanted to recapture, he said the intensity, the bonding and euphoria. I told Malcolm that in traditional Chinese medicine these are functions of the heart. If you want to recapture that, you need to feed the heart by living a life of passion, inspiration and joy. Hating everything in your life depletes the heart. The only way Malcolm could recapture the intensity and euphoria was by thinking about who he was, what his destiny was, then following it.

Ecstasy can make you aware of who you really are. It can also make you aware of whether you are living in accord with your true nature, whether you want it to or not. Ecstasy can also open the heart and generate a spiritual

Hating everything in your life depletes the heart. The only way Malcolm could recapture the intensity and euphoria was by thinking about who he was, what his destiny was, then following it.

● ● ● ● ● ● ● ●

awakening. When I mentioned this Malcolm reacted strongly. In his profession drugs were associated with criminality not spirituality. For Malcolm a spiritual experience would involve sacredness, love and communion with others. I pointed out that this was pretty close to the way ecstasy made him feel.

I ran through a program for him that would deliver the results he wanted, but he resisted. He didn't want to change his life. He felt he was in too deep, and he moved in social circles that would never permit him to suddenly become 'alternative'. He didn't want to let go of the idea that ecstasy was fun, a kind of extreme sport of the psyche. He just wanted to be high. He had tried practices that can evoke heightened states of awareness, but they didn't work for him, because he refused to look at himself and make changes. What he really wanted was a drug replacement he could turn on in an instant, but you can't turn spirituality on for a high as if it was a drug—you have to live it.

TAKING RESPONSIBILITY

If Malcolm had never tried ecstasy everything would have been fine. However, a door had been opened and the only way for him to recapture what he wanted would be to walk through and discover his soul purpose, then follow that regardless of the expectations of others. After the experiences he'd had, he *had* to be true to himself. Like many, Malcolm did not understand the responsibilities that come with drug use.

20 TOO GOOD TOO QUICK

A common mistake people make in life after drugs is trying to be too good too quick. They are totally committed and give up everything imaginable all at once. After two or three months they can't stand it, and switch from extreme virtue to extreme bingeing.

Jerry, a photographer, had been using $500 of ice per day for eighteen months, then stopped cold turkey. He became a vegetarian, gave up coffee, cigarettes, alcohol and all toxins, and had acupuncture daily at a college clinic. Two weeks into this, I asked him how long he was planning on living like that. 'Forever—it's my path now,' he said confidently. When I told him I could only have held out for a few months with that lifestyle before cracking, he seemed taken aback. He hadn't expected this response.

On drugs I had been a party person like Jerry. After a few months without drugs, purity started to feel like punishment and deprivation rather than self-development. I was so sick of being good, I needed to be really, really bad. I would binge on anything I could get my hands on. While I was bingeing it was middle finger up to everything. Afterwards I would be devastated and think I had lost all the hard work I had done. Whenever this happened, family members would make me feel even worse by saying, 'I knew you couldn't do it.' This would make me so furious. They had no idea how empty I felt and how hard it was for me to be on the virtuous path.

Some people can successfully take the path of purity and abstinence, but for others it is much harder. They need to customise their recovery strategy accordingly. In the early days after quitting speed, I felt so left out. I wanted the raging, excitement and fascination of the drug scene. Without hard drugs that feeling of something special, exotic and out of the norm was missing. Like me, Jerry was the type to crash if he stuck to that path. That would mean using ice again. I suggested he stick with the program all week, but on Fridays let himself have a reward—no rules, except no hard drugs. This gave him a much better chance of achieving his goal long term.

> Some people can successfully take the path of purity and abstinence, but for others it is much harder. They need to customise their recovery strategy accordingly.

The emphasis on the good slowly builds the organs and the intensity of bad days naturally lessens. Eventually one stiff drink feels overwhelming and the person loses interest. If you stick to the program, in time the bad day goes from excessive alcohol and excessive sex, to coffee and cake. Meanwhile, having a bad day to look forward to allows you to persevere with being good.

Many clients are surprised by the 'bad day' approach, thinking it is not spiritual. Ex-drug users need their own 'spirituality'. I have treated scores of patients who, after years of recreational drug use, felt they were polluted, so they looked to eastern spiritual purification techniques to correct this. For them life after drugs meant starting raw food diets, going on juice fasts to cleanse their systems, becoming vegetarian to lift their vibrations, taking up high-powered meditative practices and changing their name to something more spiritual. To their surprise they felt fatigued, confused, irritable and depressed, as I had done.

THE DANGERS OF GOING VEGAN

After speed I longed to be a good person. I wanted to be free of all vices and addictions, to be radiant, healthy, happy and to inspire others. I also wanted to cleanse myself of toxins so I ate fruit until lunchtime, then grains and uncooked food. Fully committed, I baked my own bread and ate no refined foods. A few months into this I was so tired I could barely move. Nothing was fun, and life was hard. I was dizzy, weak, having fainting spells and would blank out halfway through conversations.

As something was seriously wrong, I went to a practitioner of natural medicine who recommended a juice fast, so I gave up even more things. My symptoms got worse but I persevered, believing all the toxins were coming out. Then one morning instead of eating only fruit until lunchtime, I had a cooked breakfast of steak and eggs. The light-headedness vanished, my brain started working and I realised that if I continued down the vegan path, I would probably die. As soon as I changed my diet, the improvement to my health was dramatic.

Some healthy yang type people can eat fruit and fast, but ex-drug users are more likely to be unhealthy yin types who desperately need protein, nutrients, minerals, warm food and nourishment on every level. Our organs like cooked foods. If you eat cold raw foods the stomach and spleen have to 'cook' the food. This costs valuable energy you can't spare. After drugs you need to do your body a favour and give it everything it needs to make functioning as easy as possible. Life after drugs is still about substances that give the organs what they need to create altered states. This is why I always recommend high-powered supplements and herbs. They are condensed, easily digestible nutrients.

> Our organs like cooked foods. If you eat cold raw foods the stomach and spleen have to 'cook' the food. This costs valuable energy you can't spare. After drugs you need to do your body a favour and give it everything it needs to make functioning as easy as possible.

● ● ● ● ● ● ● ●

EXCESS AND DEFICIENCY

A lot of my clients have seen alternative therapists who recommend they fast and detoxify. If I take the pulse of someone who has been a drug user, it does indicate there is a toxic overload, which you could suggest fasting for. However, there is simultaneously a decline in bodily function, organs, immune system, vitality and mental functioning due to the overuse of the organs, in this situation there is excess *and* deficiency. If you go on cleansing diets and so on, you are running the risk of aggravating imbalances.

Ex-drug users are already severely depleted from the years of substance abuse, poor diet, incredible stress and anxiety. Food is life. If you take that away, you take away your life force. Even now, so many years after my drug days, I cannot go without food for longer than a few hours before feeling unsettled.

Ex-drug users are already severely depleted from the years of substance abuse, poor diet, incredible stress and anxiety. Food is life. If you take that away, you take away your life force.

● ● ● ● ● ● ● ● ●

THE POST-DRUG PULSE

Excessive hard-drug use leads to post-drug symptoms that we haven't fully understood yet. These symptoms are not straightforward. The pulse of most heavy drug users feels different to that of non-drug users. The frequency of the pulse has been altered somehow. There is a different quality present.

This post-drug quality in the pulse indicates a condition that is not able to be corrected or returned to the pre-existing frequency, as some fundamental changes have taken place. These are connected with the spiritual ramifications of drug use, so it is not about correcting symptoms anymore or detoxing, but about making permanent changes in your life.

TRANSFORM YOURSELF

Drugs are transformative substances, that is their purpose.[1] If you have used drugs in a recreational sense, you can still tap into this function afterwards.

You might as well, as it is a great way to value-add to your drug experiences. Most heavy drug users have destroyed all social expectations of them, plus all their own expectations, so it is an opportunity to let go of everything that is no longer you and develop what is really you. You can take the radical path of rebuilding yourself physically, spiritually and emotionally and emerging out of the ashes as a new person free of old conditioning. Giving up drugs is not the end, it's the beginning. That is a very exciting place to be.

Giving up drugs is not the end, it's the beginning. That is a very exciting place to be.

PART V:
RECREATIONAL DRUGS AND THE HUMAN SPIRIT

21 DRUGS AND THE DARK SIDE

Shortly after treating Malcolm, the ecstasy-loving lawyer, I saw Ralph, an innocent-looking teenager from a nice family. He went to a good school and lived a normal life, except he snorted a lot of speed every day. If he couldn't get speed he would binge drink, sniff petrol or use 'GBH' (gamma hydroxybutyrate, a central nervous system depressant).

Ralph wasn't interested in giving up drugs and didn't want to see me. From the minute he walked in he avoided eye contact and sat hunched over, staring at the floor. In recreational drug work, establishing a connection is my first task. If there is no connection between the counsellor and client, nothing will happen. So, I had to find some common ground where we had a similar interest but at the same time let him know that if he did offer any information, I would be non-judgemental.

We got into discussing the effects of different mixtures of substances. Sensing my interest, he became increasingly engaged. Just as I was congratulating myself on establishing some grounds for interaction, he straightened up and we made real eye contact. In a split second his eyes turned yellowish, feline and non-human. In that second a rush of black energy attacked me. 'Keep the fuck away' was the telepathic message.

Shock and adrenalin hit me simultaneously. Instinctively I drew on my years of training with my spiritual teacher, and my ongoing chi and martial arts training, to put myself into a meditative state of surrender to the highest source of good. I was fully present in the moment but didn't question anything. Because I had no emotion, that negative energy had no way of getting in. I kept talking casually to the boy as if nothing had happened. I could feel the presence trying to engage me, but I knew if that happened I would be on my own. So I held my position, let it be and focused only on Ralph. Finally I could feel the force dissipating, and then saw an immediate lifting in the boy's spirit. His eyes looked normal, his face opened up and some of the heaviness had gone.

Ralph hadn't noticed anything, but he did start to talk more openly about his drug experiences, concerns and problems. He wanted to know why he got certain side-effects like nausea, anger and the bad vivid dreams. Then he became curious about how I was living. He couldn't work out why I could still seem so passionate about drugs but have no interest in taking them. I talked about how I still chased those altered states through meditation, martial arts and other means. That led him to ask more questions about life after drugs. He said casually that maybe one day he would give up, and wanted to know how life was afterwards. The rest of the session went really well and Ralph left on a positive note, laughing and saying he would give me a call in ten years.

DRUGS AND NEGATIVE ENERGIES

Afterwards I sat down and tried to process what had happened. I had sensed negative energies in people before, during hands-on bodywork, but nothing like this. It was a big wake-up call. With the clients I had treated to date, it was all about giving up, learning from drugs, recapturing positive states and identifying therapeutic outcomes. I could happily chat all day about ecstasy and LSD and spirituality, but if I wanted to continue this work I was going to have to acknowledge the connection between drugs and dark forces or negative energies.

The session with Ralph also made me see that the decades of spiritual training had been preparing me for this aspect of the work. I'd had the great fortune of meeting and training under a spiritual teacher who had armed me with exactly the tools I needed to deal with the metaphysics of drugs. He'd taught me that just as the visible world has its mix of positive and negative, so too do the invisible worlds. Drug users 'open up' without knowing it, then charge into invisible worlds totally unprepared. Like naive tourists stumbling into the bad part of town, they have no idea where they are heading.

> Drug users 'open up' without knowing it, then charge into invisible worlds totally unprepared. Like naive tourists stumbling into the bad part of town, they have no idea where they are heading.

CONTINUING THE JOURNEY

I began my spiritual training a few years after the rainbow bridge workshop. I had no idea what I was doing with that technique but the great feeling of energy moving through me was addictive. Transcendental meditation was the next thing I tried, but I couldn't relax, because I felt I had to hide my past. So I kept going with my daily tai-chi and chi-gung instead. I did join a few more meditation groups but nothing really clicked for me. Then I went to a meditation seminar that did. The teacher was Indian. He had a turban and long white beard, and his presence put me completely at ease. I wasn't the least bit worried about what others in the room would think of me. The teacher led us in a group meditation, which was a blissful and sacred experience. Afterwards he asked if anyone had any questions. I put up my hand and asked if we were allowed to drink alcohol.

The minute the words left my mouth I regretted it. I had done the wrong thing, again. Just as my self-esteem started to plummet, his face lit up and to the surprise of everyone he enthusiastically shouted, 'Of course you can.' He started talking about how much he liked red wine. He seemed to think this was really funny and slapped his knees and laughed loudly to himself. I felt such relief at his response, I knew I could trust him.

Meeting him had a profound impact on me and from then on whenever he was in Australia I would travel to wherever he was. He talked about spirits not allowed to incarnate on the earthly plane and ghosts. He knew I was doing martial arts training and described how he had seen people break rocks without touching them and perform other supernatural feats. This was such a feast for me. Here was someone respectable who had never taken drugs, yet was speaking about worlds I had thought only drugs could access.

There was always a sense that things were happening. Even if we were sitting in a suburban fish and chip shop somewhere, there was the kind of buzz around him I thought you could only get by snorting cocaine in a fantastic nightclub. He gradually became my mentor and teacher. He taught me to instantly access altered states and how to avoid the influence of the dark forces. His belief was that heaven and hell exist at the same time in the same place, and once 'opened up' you were exposed to both.

He said that meditation was neither good nor bad, it was how you applied it that determined the outcome. You didn't just 'open up' as you do on drugs. You used mantras and actively called upon love, the divine and higher powers to direct the experience. The idea was to align with the highest source of good—that would naturally keep the negative forces at bay. My spiritual teacher believed certain people are at a higher risk of exposure to negative energies than others. According to him this included therapists who worked with energy techniques, ambulance drivers, hospital workers and drug users.

He, of course, had no knowledge of recreational drugs and I had been avoiding mentioning that part of my past to him. When I hesitantly made some reference to it he was not interested in my past, but in where I wanted to go.

A PATIENT WITH A DIFFERENCE

Several years after I started my training with him, he must have decided it was time for some practical sessions. He invited me to come to Malaysia. At that time I was still doing energy healing using acupuncture and the bodywork, and would constantly use reference books. So I headed off to Malaysia with a massage table and my books. I set up a room in a hotel where I could treat patients under the supervision of my teacher.

My first patient was having difficulty walking as she had trouble controlling her lower legs and feet. When I asked how it had happened, the translator hesitated for a moment then said the woman had had a spell put on her. I thought I had misheard but the translator explained the woman had made eye contact with someone else's husband, so the man's wife had gone to the village witchdoctor to get a curse put on her.

I stared blankly at one of my books, desperately trying to process this information. I was way out of my depth. My teacher simply stroked his beard, nodded and smiled. I decided the best approach would be to just keep busy, so I took her pulse and looked at her tongue, but didn't get much from that. Then I asked her to get on the massage table, so I could begin the high-energy bodywork and acupuncture. As soon as I began to work with the needles and my hands, things changed. I was now relying on intuition, gut instinct and faith. It wasn't long before I sensed her energy field, which was pleasant and warm. But I could also sense, overlying it, an energy grid that was cold, hard and foreign. Intuitively I knew this was the problem. I used my training in meditation and tai-chi to put myself in a meditative state. I could feel the energetic guidance and support of my teacher and I engaged with the 'grid'.

Focusing on putting pressure on the grid, I used psychic energy to drive to the core of it. I didn't let go until I could feel a dissolving of that energy. A stream of colours and images shot through me. I had a sense of matter and 'will' disintegrating and dispersing. I followed it and kept chasing the remnants. After about forty-five minutes her energy field became clear and a renewed flow of energy began. My client felt heat and tingling in her legs and she could move her big toe again. Her face looked different too. As she walked across the room her ability to control her feet had definitely improved. She was delighted.

There was no logical explanation for what had happened, but at the same time everything made perfect sense. There had been some intelligence in her that was not her. It was my first experience of trusting my spiritual and chi training, as well as the techniques I had learned at college. There weren't any more clients with curses after that, but in some patients I sensed a negative energy or entity. As soon as I united with the energy field of the patient, it seemed to transfer to me. After some of these cases, heaviness, nausea and an almost uncontrollable aggravation would overwhelm me. I felt like screaming and smashing things. My teacher said it was a spiritual attack or invasion. I felt uneasy, immediately picturing the worst scenes from horror movies, but he said it was good training. It would strengthen me spiritually, because I would be forced to learn how to deal with it.

22 THE LOWER REALMS

From that very first meditation my teacher had told us that it was a conscious experience of the subconscious, so we would become aware of our unresolved issues. After each session unpleasant emotions or memories would come forward. He suggested we form a meditation group of our own, to continue the practice and discuss our experiences, so we immediately organised a venue and group, and met regularly.

We really got into it and decided to do weekend meditation retreats. The first one was a great success. For me it was a blissful few days, but as I was driving home an acidic, bitter feeling permeated my body and mind. By the time I arrived home it had turned to anger and resentment. I was sure my partner was blocking my progress and everything was her fault. I stomped in the door and refused even to say hello. She asked what was going on so I accused her of picking a fight with me. Then the cycle of emotionality started. It led to days of accusations and confusion, until we reached the point where we talked about splitting up. I brought this up at our next group meeting but no one had any idea what we were dealing with.

DRUG-FREE RAVING

I did not understand what was being released, or how to process it. The meditative experience was so blissful I thought it was the ultimate high. I felt so good my immediate instinct was to go out partying to clubs, dance parties or raves to keep the 'high' going. I would choose venues that had psychedelic atmospheres with incredible light shows and a group consciousness of ecstasy. There I would join in with hundreds of people who were dancing to trance beats and bonding with each other.

I remember one night going to a huge dance party of nearly a thousand people. I made my way to the front where the DJ was. The surge of energy behind me directed at the DJ was incredible and I turned to face the crowd. Now I was soaking it up from everyone. It was a powerful pulsating roar throbbing in my veins. Without thinking I flipped back into a drug-world behaviour. I needed to be higher. I put myself into the meditative state again and drew on that energy as well. It was pretty mind-blowing.

We used to do this thing in the 1970s called eye-locking, where a few of us who were tripping on LSD would 'transfer' the trip to a friend who had not taken acid. You could easily trigger the state in a willing person. That night I was opening up my energy field to allow the communal drug highs of all those people, as well as the meditative high, to merge.

The next day I felt really ill. I vomited and couldn't get out of bed. I had no idea why as I had only had water to drink. When I asked my teacher about it, he wanted to know what I thought I was doing, then launched into a long explanation about how raves and clubs are highly attractive to spirits and entities. Because so many people there were opened up through drugs, their boundaries were dissolving. Energetic exchanges and merges were occurring without anyone realising it. It was an energetic free-for-all. In those places, being 'opened up' by meditation was the same as being 'opened up' by drugs. I didn't have the years of training or understanding to protect myself. Spiritual contamination was the result.

> Because so many people at the rave were opened up through drugs, their boundaries were dissolving. Energetic exchanges and merges were occurring without anyone realising it. It was an energetic free-for-all.

At the time I reacted against the idea of being contaminated. It wasn't that far past my drug days and in my mind feeling high was still connected with clubs, bars and partying and I didn't see what the problem was. He did offer to do a cleansing for me though. Afterwards I felt on top of the world, so there was something in what he said.

DRUGS AND HELLISH EXPERIENCES

As I continued working with my teacher I learned more about the spirits and entities of the lower realms. I also discovered what became my favourite book, the *Autobiography of a Yogi*, written by the spiritual luminary Yogananda. He mentioned that although pure-minded humans can glimpse good spirit beings or worlds, drug use allows access to astral hells.[1] This is why many scriptures forbid drug use. That caught my attention but I didn't want to think about it in relation to my own past. I preferred to believe drugs had only shown me beautiful, sacred beings and wonderful worlds. But the truth was that there was a much darker side as well.

In traditional Chinese medicine, a belief in spirits and demons is part of the underpinning philosophy. There are acupuncture 'ghost points' to treat spirit invasion. It is said that spirit-like creatures, some good and some evil, wander in the world of spirit.[2] In certain situations or circumstances they become visible in the material world. Ongoing drug use is one of these situations. One first century Chinese medical text states that using hemp (the cannabis plant) to excess makes one see monsters, but over a long period of time it can enable the user to establish contact with spirits.[3] The connection between drugs and spiritual invasion was there but I didn't apply this to my own experiences, until after that session with Ralph and the attack by some sort of entity.

> I preferred to believe drugs had only shown me beautiful, sacred beings and wonderful worlds. But the truth was that there was a much darker side as well.

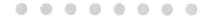

HASHISH, JAIL AND SPIRITS

When I was about twenty-two my best friend got busted and sent to jail. I was out when the police came, otherwise I would have been arrested instead. Feeling guilt-ridden, I wanted to show my support and loyalty. Risking my own safety to bring him drugs seemed like the way to do it, so I smuggled hash into the prison.

After lights-out that night he smoked a few pipes, then he sat on the bed looking forward to just drifting away. But instead of bliss, a malignant presence joined him. Before he could come to terms with this, a powerful blow to the chest sent him flying back across the bed. He got the fright of his life. He fumbled for his lighter, but there was nothing in the room. His hands shook so much the shadows started shifting into sinister forms, so he quickly extinguished the lighter and spent the rest of the night bolt upright on the bed, terrified.

He told me all of this after he got out. We were both stoned at the time. Usually I loved supernatural stories, but this one made me fearful and anxious. My speed use was taking its toll. I was getting confused and subconsciously knew a dark element had entered our world. I was scared that talking about these things would draw me further under its spell. It is fun to discuss aliens and ghosts when you are sure of yourself, but when you are mentally off-balance it doesn't take much for them to come and get you. I wasn't feeling good about life anymore. The tension was mounting. Something had to change, and a few weeks later it did.

THE DAY I DECIDED TO DIE

My friend and I had just done eighteen hours on speed and were coming down. I could feel the familiar empty frustration, the anxiety and the paranoia. I felt like crying. We were driving aimlessly trying to avoid the post-speed low. It must have been a Sunday because as we approached a church, I could see a group of well-dressed people standing outside laughing and talking. I felt a stab of envy at the ease with which they could communicate with each other.

At the same time they represented everything I didn't want—the straight world of routine.

Standing near the church gate was a middle-aged woman wearing a tailored coat, sensible shoes and a lifetime of repression and judgement. Our eyes met momentarily as we passed, and a look of utter distaste involuntarily crossed her face. My long hair and graffiti-covered van obviously represented everything she didn't want and I had the startling realisation that I could never go back to that normal world even if I wanted to because they didn't want me. Loss and hopelessness washed over me, along with real anger. I didn't care if I was an outsider, because I didn't want the world of Sundays and happiness. I belonged to the drug world, and I was going to take drugs until I died.

As soon as this thought entered my head I felt an incredible sense of relief. The frightening part was how right that choice seemed. Even in my anger and desolation, I knew without a doubt that some force was encouraging me to take the path towards death. Its presence was chillingly tangible. I told myself I didn't care. I turned the car around and went to score more drugs. Then we went back to the squat and had our own Sunday special of some high-quality speed. Within minutes I knew this was the world I belonged in. I would have as many more years of highs as I could then finish everything with one final shot. There were no other options. It was the first day of the end of my life.

> Even in my anger and desolation, I knew without a doubt that some force was encouraging me to take the path towards death. Its presence was chillingly tangible. I told myself I didn't care. I turned the car around and went to score more drugs.

EMBRACING DESTRUCTION

That day marked the start of a much darker period of my life. The positive, life-affirming drug escapades and the hippie dream had come to an end. I couldn't see the purpose in life anymore. This affected me on every level. My appearance changed, my taste in music changed and my attitude changed to one of defeat.

At that stage I was dropping by my parents' house to use the shower and occasionally to eat. On my next visit I found a box of prescription medication for my mother's migraines on a bench. It was a powerful morphine-based medicine. Without a second thought, I opened the box and took the lot. It was good stuff. I went to my old room, put on a record, and lay there semi-conscious and numb. I felt quite good, but must have looked terrible.

My mother realised what I had done and came into my room. She was utterly devastated. She managed to control herself and said, 'I know you are going to die, you are not going to make it, I'm going to lose my son.' I should have felt compassion or sorrow but I was detached and cold. In that moment that same feeling of external support came in to back me up.

From then on every time I chose destruction that feeling of back-up became stronger. Everyone needs support. Supporting those who can't be good may be the role of the fallen angels. I don't believe people are born bad. When I worked with street kids I saw first-hand the development of criminality. They were great kids, but they got trapped in negative situations. After a while it is easier to give in to it than fight. Each day I felt as if I was being lured closer and closer to the dark. Support for this direction grew. It gave me power and made me feel I was not alone. It comforted me.

23 MAGIC MUSHROOMS

Moving to Australia drew me out of the vortex. When I arrived in the hippie commune I found myself surrounded by people doing life-affirming things. They all took drugs, but the hippie drugs: marijuana, mushrooms and LSD. There was none of the despair and destruction of the speed scene. I desperately wanted to be like them but was so destroyed from the speed I couldn't connect with what was going on around me. I needed a magical, mystical ceremony to initiate me back into life, and the only way I knew how to get that was through psychedelic drugs. Seeking an experience as earthy and spiritual as possible, I knew the drug had to be magic mushrooms. I wrote in my diary:

> I am in a forest looking over the valley. The magic mushrooms are brewing within me pulsating, alive and giving out energy. I feel it knocking at the door. It wants to be set free.
>
> I let myself be drawn by a massive spiral into the depths of my body. Then, I forget everything, become totally passive, let go, surrender and fall. Everything is spinning around me. The world is sliding past; faster, quicker. I give myself over to ecstasy. I watch the stars racing past. I know that I know nothing anymore, still I know everything. Everything is so clear and easy.
>
> Now it is happening, the energy is gripping my soul. It compresses it, tears it and sparks fly from it. I explode out of my body, out of the world, and I am

dragged along a vortex. And there it is: the peak. I arrive at Nirvana. Peace. A soft and velvety land, framed by pink flowers. In the distance there are mountains, peaceful and welcoming. There are beings, foreign but familiar. I have met them before, so they are not strangers to me. Ah, I remember them, but I don't know why I remember them. I don't know these beings yet I remember them.

It is a beautiful world, like a dream, but it is real. I am welcomed as a visitor and I feel the land. It is eternal and timeless. It is totally different to what I knew until now but not new either. I will return to live in harmony with this land, I know it for sure. The land makes me feel secure, it is my home. I will return after I have travelled the earth in human form long enough. I'm not doing a trip at the moment. It is when I leave this land and return to reality that the trip begins.

THE TRUTH DRUG

I wrote that diary entry while I was on the mushrooms. In those days I considered magic mushrooms to be a truth drug. What you feel about yourself on them is what you really feel. With the psychedelic drugs you can't hide from what you are. Our unconscious beliefs shape our actions. The mushrooms allow direct access to these beliefs. I knew that if I could embrace life on a mushroom trip, I could embrace life in reality. Because I felt so welcomed and had such a sense of belonging and nurturing, that trip confirmed my intent to live. Psychedelic drugs can catalyse consciousness, speeding up processes that are already present.[1] That trip probably had the same impact that years of therapy might have had.

MUSHROOMS AND SHAMANISM

Magic mushrooms have been used for thousands of years, for ritual rather than recreational reasons. The renowned shaman María Sabina said that the further you go into the world of the mushrooms, the more things are seen and known. Your past and future are accessible together as a single entity.[2] This ability to access knowledge, travel to other realities and interact with beings after consuming psychedelic drugs seems inexplicable. However, this property of the mushrooms needs to be respected as it is in traditional cultures that have shamans.

THE BAD MUSHROOM TRIP

I have no explanation for what happened on that mushroom trip. It did have a positive outcome, but using mushrooms or any other psychedelic drugs in the state I was in was probably not a good idea. It could so easily have turned against me and then I don't know what I would have done.

A friend of mine recently recounted one of his mushroom trips that started with a suffocating darkness. He focused on trying not to panic and on continuing to breathe. Then a new reality opened up—a jarring, threatening, alien place, where he was instantly confronted by a hideous being with large black dead reptilian eyes. He was not welcome there. The being transmitted this message very clearly. He had to get out, so he crashed back into his body shaken and exhausted. It was so real yet so far beyond rational explanation that he couldn't speak about what had happened for over two years.

I have had many patients who took large doses of mushrooms, then developed psychosis, or else some part of them got stuck in an altered state. They had seen the world in a different way and it did not return to normal afterwards. Not returning could have been my fate.

MYSTICAL EXPERIENCES

Magic mushrooms are sometimes described as entheogens, which means 'becoming divine within'. Some researchers believe that religions developed as a result of the non-ordinary states of consciousness generated by these psychoactive substances.[3] After my experiences with magic mushrooms and other drugs including mescaline, I can certainly understand how that theory emerged. You do feel you have been granted access to another realm and the beings inhabiting those places seem absolutely real. Even the most recent mainstream psychedelic drug study, evaluating the acute and longer-term psychological effects of the magic mushroom, found that it 'can occasion mystical-type experiences having substantial and sustained personal meaning and spiritual significance'.[4]

24 DRUGS AND SPIRITUAL INVASION

According to traditional Chinese medicine, drugs use the organs as a platform to work from. Each organ has a spiritual as well as physical and emotional function. The organs can also be gateways to the unseen worlds. The spleen is a key organ in magic mushroom trips, because it is responsible for digestion on both the physical level, which explains the vomiting frequently experienced prior to the onset of a trip, and 'digesting' what is happening on the mental level. The spleen governs our physical boundaries, and those between the concrete and abstract, or the visible and invisible worlds. So, this is where doorways are opened and other dimensions possibly accessed.

Drug consumption damages the organs and this can have negative spiritual repercussions. There are spiritual influences around us all the time, but when we are so solidly in matter, we don't notice them. In physics, matter and energy are interchangeable: matter is simply slowed-down energy.[1] In traditional Chinese medicine we use the terms 'yin' and 'yang' for matter and energy. The visible world is condensed, heavy and yin, or matter. The spiritual world, which is ethereal and constantly shifting, is yang, or energy. Drugs disintegrate the boundaries between the physical and spiritual worlds and allow the human energy field to become permeable.

Once we alter the relationship between energy and matter (by using drugs, for example) and become more energy, we can open to energetic exchange or invasion. In that session with Ralph I believe I crossed paths with an inhabitant of the astral hells. It was a negative entity that wanted to experience human life and it had temporarily

Drugs disintegrate the boundaries between the physical and spiritual worlds and allow the human energy field to become permeable.

● ● ● ● ● ● ● ● ●

taken hold of him. It did not want me preventing this. I am sure that Ralph had no idea about this. I believe it is something that happens accidentally.

I was still reluctant to think about this too deeply, though. Then a wave of new clients came in worried about having attracted spirits from their drug-taking. They talked about feeling heavy energy 'stuck' to them or entities following them around, so I had to re-examine my own past as well as drawing upon my spiritual studies. Everything my teacher had said about the astral worlds and negative entities took on a new significance. It also brought up more memories that I had been holding down for years.

DRUGS, DEALING AND DARKNESS

One of the strongest memories I recalled was from my dealing days in Amsterdam. I had gone there with my best friend. We were getting some gear to run back to Germany to sell. My friend was with the money and the supplier on one side of town, while I had gone with a middleman to pick the gear up. He had driven me to a really bad area of the city. We parked near a dilapidated old factory. I followed him through a warren of corridors until he opened a door and told me to wait there while he got the stuff.

It was a huge empty room, with dirty light filtering through the smashed windows. Someone was lying on the floor. I hoped he was alive. Another two guys were sitting in the far corner staring blankly. They didn't acknowledge me. There was a chair just inside the door. I sat there for what seemed like a very long time. Nothing happened. Then I sensed movement in my peripheral vision. I turned to see a group of large black reptilian-beings creeping up the wall. The only thought in my head was that they were more alive than the humans in the room. I told myself it was a hallucination, but I never hallucinated on speed.

One of those reptiles made eye contact with me. In my past experiences of encountering unpleasant entities while on LSD or other drugs, there was normally shock from one or both parties and the feeling that they wanted me out of their world. This time there was no surprise on either side, which meant I was not unknown to them. Our vibrational frequencies must have been approaching a match. Subconsciously I knew if I didn't make some changes this was the world I would be heading towards—not necessarily a world of alien reptiles, but a world of coldness, bitterness, indifference and cruelty. I was probably halfway there already.

Drugs are not a nice business to be involved in. The further into that world I went, the more unpleasant the interactions became. Each day there was a little bit less hope and goodness, and the doors to the dark worlds opened up a fraction more. I saw bad things, real and unreal. I felt heavier and heavier, as if something was physically weighing me down, but there seemed no way out of it, no turning back. I think my friend and I both knew how it was going to end.

POST-DRUG PURIFICATION

It is this feeling of heaviness that subconsciously drives many ex-drug users to fasting and purging after they quit. You feel as if you want to cleanse yourself of something, but it may well be something non-physical that you have acquired without knowing it. Spiritual techniques are required to remove it.

Fasting is not recommended because it weakens your defences, and the sense of spiritual invasion can become more dominant. The focus needs to be on strengthening yourself on every level. Collect as many physical reminders of attracting the good into your life as possible. Surround yourself with holy pictures, and sacred books and objects.

Replenish your organs to build up strength and willpower. When your organs are deficient it is very difficult to control fear, and therefore attacks can worsen. Get professionally prescribed Chinese herbs and take them regularly as this impacts on your psychological, emotional and spiritual health. Practice chi-gung or a martial art, and do a daily meditation dedicated to the light to neutralise the influence of negative energies.

LEAVING THE DARK PATH

Back in Germany I had no idea about any of this. I just knew that everything in my life was wrong. I was getting weaker by the day, I was taking more drugs, had less sleep, less food, no positivity. Aggression and anger dominated. There was nothing to feed my heart. Once I got to Australia I just wanted to put all of that behind me. Thinking about the past made me sick and confused. I didn't want to acknowledge the things I had seen or done. I also felt guilty because I got out of Germany and my friends didn't.

I felt like I had abandoned my comrades, especially my best friend, and I couldn't forgive myself for that, as my relationship with him was the closest I had. We had lived together, explored other universes together and were closer than brothers. Sadly, by the time I left we had both gone so far down the dark path that I didn't even say goodbye.

> I just knew that everything in my life was wrong. I was getting weaker by the day, I was taking more drugs, had less sleep, less food, no positivity. Aggression and anger dominated. There was nothing to feed my heart.

Later, after my health and outlook had improved, I was too scared to make contact, worried he would drag me back down again, or reject me or attack me for running away. All the madness we had been through made sense when we were on drugs, but without the drugs I couldn't make sense of any of it.

I found out recently that he continued taking hard drugs and drinking and became bitter, alienated and depressed. Eight years after I left, he died in a clinic. It was the news I had been dreading. The shock and sadness still haven't left me and I don't know if they ever will. The drug journey shouldn't end this way for anyone. His death was a reminder for me of how easily it can go wrong. Ongoing drug use weakens the spirit to such a level that you can give up on life and die. For the rest of my life his death will remind me how dangerous the drug path is. To empower people and give them a reason to live, we must strengthen their spirit. To do this we need to change our approach to drugs and drug users to stop more deaths. We are spiritual beings, and drug use is ultimately about spirit.

> To empower people and give them a reason to live, we must strengthen their spirit. To do this we need to change our approach to drugs and drug users to stop more deaths.
> We are spiritual beings, and drug use is ultimately about spirit.

● ● ● ● ● ● ● ●

PART VI:
DRUGS AND PSYCHOSIS

25 PSYCHOSIS

As the clients with metaphysical drug issues began tapering off, I got a call from a mother wanting to book her 'psychotic' daughter in for a six-week program.

Sharon was twenty-three and had taken so much speed that, according to her mother, she was 'totally crazy'. She had become obsessed with a well-known pop star—she dressed the way he did, and was convinced she was in contact with him. The mother had booked her into a rehab clinic. Sharon retaliated by using speed the minute she got out. After her third time in rehab Sharon did stop using drugs, and her mother thought the problem was solved. She was looking forward to life going back to normal, but Sharon maintained her obsessions and became increasingly bitter and frustrated with her parents. They feared Sharon was going to have to be institutionalised.

I was apprehensive about the case. From her mother's description I would be facing someone with active but absent eyes, who answered questions I hadn't asked, who constantly fidgeted or laughed for no reason, someone who felt threatened by me and might attack: someone like I had been.

By treating a psychotic client, I would be putting myself on the line psychologically, because psychosis makes you so 'opened up' you are also extremely insightful. You can read others' thoughts and sense who people really are. If Sharon was in the state her mother described, she would know straight away if there was something imbalanced in me. And if there was, my ability to help her would be drastically reduced.

A few weeks later Sharon arrived and to my great relief she was nowhere near as 'crazy' as her mother thought. Sure, she was wearing eccentric clothes, was obsessed by some pop star, and was moody and disinterested, but that wasn't madness. I thought she looked great, unique, a real individual.

Sharon said the problem was her parents. They had taken her to see a psychiatrist who had diagnosed Sharon as psychotic and prescribed medication. The psychiatrist also suggested her parents firmly oppose Sharon's delusional activities and ideas. This created ongoing confrontation and made Sharon even more reactive. Due to her drug use, Sharon didn't have enough flexibility (yin) to move to an alternative position, so any comment that challenged her would naturally lead to confrontation or denial.

I counsel many devastated and frustrated parents who say their child is 'psychotic' from drugs but won't admit it. I know how those kids feel. You know something is not right with your mind but you can't move out of your position. So, you have to deny it, or else you will become it, you will be mad. Denial is a survival strategy, because in denial there is hope.

Sharon had already used prescription medications recreationally, as many drug users do, and had become very good at working out what combinations deliver what results. She decided that if her parents wanted her medicated she would be. She independently went off to several doctors, reported differing symptoms and managed to get painkillers, tranquillisers and medications for attention deficit disorder. She was taking handfuls of pills. It was no wonder none of her symptoms had gone. Her attitude was that since she was a 'stuff-up' she might as well spend the rest of her life medicated.

LOSING CONTROL

The minute she said this, I remembered some more things about my past. I too had reached the stage where I decided I would have to be medicated for life. My speed hangovers were getting worse and I had started getting noticeably weird. I was having trouble talking, was unwilling to participate in anything, and felt annoyed and empty. The psychological confusion was the worst part, though.

By the time I got to Australia the mental confusion became unbearable. I often couldn't tell the difference between what people said and the static and sounds circling in my own head. It was scary. I went to elaborate lengths to avoid being in a confined space with people for any length of time because if someone confronted me I didn't know what I would do. My secret fear was of publicly losing control and becoming violent.

Right at the height of this period of confusion, I needed to get permanent residency. Some straight middle-aged friends of my parents knew a member of parliament who could help, so a meeting was arranged with myself and the member of parliament at their place. I arrived on time but the MP was running late, so I ended up sitting in the lounge with my parents' friends for what seemed like hours. It wasn't long before I started to feel on edge. They were making polite conversation, but I couldn't settle, my mind was all over the place. The stakes were high because without permanent residency I would be going back to Germany and that meant jail.

The pressure made everything worse. My mouth was as dry as dust but I was too scared to drink anything because I had the shakes. My head started buzzing with disconnected thoughts and I was getting more and more worried that I wouldn't be able to distinguish between my thoughts and reality. The occasional pauses in conversation, which were probably about ten seconds in length, felt like hours. Silence was dangerous ground for me. At the next pause, I panicked. Thinking my host had been talking about sewing, I responded, but she hadn't said anything. There was a horrible silence.

> I went to elaborate lengths to avoid being in a confined space with people for any length of time because if someone confronted me I didn't know what I would do. My secret fear was of publicly losing control and becoming violent.

Just then the MP arrived. Getting up to greet him released most of the tension, as it took the focus off me. There was a quick conversation and a handshake, and the friends of my parents provided a reference for me. The MP left with me close behind him. I was ready to collapse from the stress of trying to hold it together.

The MP phoned me several days later to let me know that my application would be approved. Had I known he would call, I would have medicated myself with alcohol or pills, so that I could function. He asked me some innocuous question to be polite. Because he was important, I panicked. I knew I was required to express my gratitude but couldn't work out how. I felt myself becoming more and more hyper.

In desperation I started babbling about Christmas and other festivities and laughed lots in an attempt to appear positive. There was silence at the other end. He asked me if I was mad. I was so shocked I couldn't speak. He hung up. That was the first time someone had accused me outright of being mad. For the rest of the day I had to chain-smoke cigarettes and drink to regain some balance.

THE PRESCRIPTION

That episode was the final straw. I was living in a minefield and I couldn't take it anymore. The alcohol and pills weren't doing enough to control my mind. Maybe the MP was right, maybe I was mad. Perhaps I had ruined my life with drugs. If so I might as well get some heavy medication and stay on it. I wanted to be able to talk, have a normal conversation on the telephone and to socialise. I wanted something to control my mind. Like Sharon, I had abused enough pharmaceutical drugs to understand their qualities. I thought I needed tranquillisers. After much careful rehearsal of what symptoms to present, I made an appointment with a doctor.

My underlying anxiety escalated as soon as I saw him. I told him all about my high stress levels, my inability to relax and my feelings of claustrophobia, and I suggested that perhaps I needed something to settle my mind. My voice was shaky and I had spoken a little too fast. I was sure he had seen through me. Before I could stop myself I laughed hysterically. Then came a frenetic jumble of words. I felt dizzy and frightened as the doctor had the power to put me away and I was acting like a lunatic.

Thankfully his phone rang. After a brief conversation, he picked up his pad and wrote out a prescription for powerful tranquillisers. As he passed it to me, he looked me directly in the eyes and said, 'You only have one life— don't waste it.' I left confused but in some strange way uplifted. I did get the prescription filled but couldn't take it for days. When I did, it didn't feel right. I didn't want to go through the rest of my life numbed and medicated, but I didn't want to remain how I was either. At the time it seemed there were no other options.

BUILDING THE BODY

Sharon said she was choosing to be medicated for life, but I knew she didn't really want to be. No one does. You do so because you feel stuck, frustrated and hopeless. In my mind, Sharon's major symptom was seriously depleted organs so my focus was on rebuilding them. Once you have physical balance and strength you have mental balance and strength, and a reference to centre yourself. From there you can have options. You develop a healthy relationship with your desires, and obsessions are more likely to resolve themselves.

I organised an intensive program of counselling, acupuncture, deep tissue massage, exercise, tai-chi and regular meals to build the organs and give Sharon a sense of physical and emotional centre. She was used to the rehab centres and all the patient games that arise where people are placed in these centres against their wishes. But I had chosen therapists who could understand her position and wouldn't react to anything she did, and I had a health professional monitor her medication.

Despite her verbal resistance Sharon turned up for all the sessions, and followed all the recommendations. At the end of the six weeks because she was free of us, she celebrated by taking handfuls of pills. Her parents could see a marked change in her as the routine, improved diet and powerful nutritional supplements had allowed some physical healing. They were worried she would fall back into her addictive behaviour. I advised them to let her be. Free choice is an important part of getting off drugs. Ideally you don't oppose people's choices as it leads to reaction. If Sharon wanted to change she would do so in her own time. She had all the puzzle pieces, she had been introduced to her chi or inner energy, she had felt balance and she had options. It was up to her now. Six months later her mother phoned to say she couldn't believe the difference in Sharon. She ate three meals a day, kept the tai-chi going and was no longer abusing medications.

> Free choice is an important part of getting off drugs. Ideally you don't oppose people's choices as it leads to reaction. If Sharon wanted to change she would do so in her own time. She had all the puzzle pieces, she had been introduced to her chi or inner energy, she had felt balance and she had options. It was up to her now.

● ● ● ● ● ● ● ●

26 PSYCHOSIS AND SUPPRESSED ISSUES

It was a bit of a shock to find someone like Sharon had been labelled psychotic, when she was practically normal. It didn't occur to me until later that I was measuring 'normal' against how I had been.

Harry, a lively, energetic 29-year-old, walked in to the consultation room stating he was psychotic. He seemed quite comfortable saying this out loud. As I discovered later, he was self-diagnosed. After a recent three-day ice binge something weird had happened to him. He woke up badly hungover and concerned that he wouldn't be able to go to work the following day. Needing to do something active but monotonous to help him get focused and keep the symptoms down, he decided to paint his bedroom.

Knowing the exact shade of green he wanted, he went off to a hardware store to buy some paint. Harry found the paint and was heading to the cash registers when he ran into a relative who began asking what he was doing there and why he wanted green paint. In her opinion cream or white would have been more appropriate. This particular relative had always been on his case and her negative reaction really irritated him, so he started arguing with her. Other shoppers stood around watching what quickly became a yelling match.

Feeling a tap on his shoulder from a stern-faced security guard, Harry immediately knew something was horribly wrong. He felt a physical shift or jolt, his knees went weak and he needed to urinate. The guard's voice sounded distorted. The man was asking him what he was doing, but Harry couldn't answer. He turned to his relative to help explain, but realised there was no one there. He was so shaken he dropped the paint and ran out of the shop.

Before going to the paint store, Harry felt all over the place. He couldn't settle and was on the verge of vomiting. He could feel static crackling around him. On the drive to the store everything outside the car was either speeding up or slowing down, sometimes both at once. Things got worse in the shop. Noises were echoing and crashing about in his head. He just wanted to get the paint and get out of there. 'Seeing' his relative stirred him up, and his anger became uncontrollable.

YIN AND YANG

I knew exactly how Harry felt. Every symptom he described was all too familiar, so while he was speaking, I drew on my own memories of being in that state. I wasn't using a verbal listening skill as much as an emotional listening skill.

When I studied counselling we were taught to listen sympathetically to clients, but I wanted more for my clients, I wanted them to *feel* hope, as hope is the first step to healing. One way to feel hope is to be with someone who has been through what you have, and has made it successfully out the other side.

If I understand the client emotionally based on my own experience, they don't feel so alone. They can safely reveal their painful secrets, the things they can't make sense of and things they are confused about. This only works if I am completely with them, yet grounded so nothing shakes me. To do this I need deep roots, which come from a lifestyle of regular tai-chi, meditation and exercise, and strong organs. Initially I was a bit reluctant to go 'out there', in case I was not able to return to centre as this is what psychosis is. But I went a bit further with each client and the roots held firm.

When Harry finished describing his symptoms, he said he couldn't believe he had argued with someone who wasn't there, and thought this meant he was psychotic and in need of permanent medication. In traditional Chinese medicine, he had experienced a temporary imbalance of body and mind. In traditional Chinese medicine the mind is pure energy (yang). The body is matter (yin). The body holds the mind in safe boundaries. Drugs disrupt the balance between body and mind, and so the mind is freed from the control of the body. Once this happens all kinds of suppressed material can come freely to the conscious mind.

Harry's episode was due to his extended speed and ice use. He had reached the point of imbalance where matter could no longer hold down a memory. We talked about the interaction with his relative as having possibly represented an unresolved issue from the past. Harry's biggest concern was that it would happen again.

> In traditional Chinese medicine the mind is pure energy (yang). The body is matter (yin). The body holds the mind in safe boundaries. Drugs disrupt the balance between body and mind, and so the mind is freed from the control of the body.

I was sure that if he made a few changes in his lifestyle he would never have another

psychotic episode and suggested he view the incident as a sign that change was on the horizon and his drug days were drawing to a close. This episode was an indicator that he had gone beyond the point where he could control the side-effects. I recommended specific Chinese raw herbs to treat the underlying organ imbalances, but the bigger picture was the opportunity to utilise this episode beneficially. Harry had experienced first-hand the consequences of suppressing issues, and could now embark on a therapy program to release his issues and improve his life on many levels.

DON'T SUPPRESS YOUR ISSUES

Heavy drug use can release suppressed issues. If this happens it is best to get some therapy and process these as soon as possible. Doing this while you are young, and have the energy and time, is highly recommended. Otherwise suppressed issues will come forward later in life. Death is the final separation

Heavy drug use can release suppressed issues. If this happens it is best to get some therapy and process these as soon as possible.

of body (yin) and mind (yang). As it draws closer, yin and yang can begin separating. If the yin is declining and yang is dominant, it creates a state similar to psychosis. In nursing homes I have noticed many elderly people 'losing it' in the way that psychotic drug users do.

My mother ended up in a dementia ward with other elderly people with the same condition. The suffering was terrible. My mother, who was careful about what she said and how she presented herself, was arguing with and screaming at people who weren't there. Her language was so foul I was shocked. She was trapped in that terrible state until her death. She was of the generation that had no concept of dealing with issues. It made me aware of how much in her life was unresolved and how important it is to deal with this when you can.

Drug use can create serious pain. However, it is also a perfect opportunity to face the consequences of living unaware in your youth while you still have the opportunity to change. What Harry had gone through could change his future by inspiring him to live in awareness from that point on.

27 PSYCHOSIS, CHAOS AND LOGIC

Unlike Harry, I didn't see people who weren't there—or not that I know of. It was the auditory delusions that got to me. Hearing voices is usually considered evidence of serious mental imbalance. However, research shows plenty of normal people also hear voices, most commonly calling their name. In a recent study over fifty percent of normal subjects reported this.[1] Hearing voices seems to have been part of human behavior since our earliest history, but is inexplicable from the mainstream scientific or medical perspective. There is some evidence that if you use recreational drugs, hearing voices, getting tapped on the shoulder and other such phenomena dramatically increase.

CHAOS

The voices I heard were not telling me what to do, they were commenting negatively on my actions. My response was to do whatever I could to make them go away. The problem was, I never knew when it was going to happen. In my first drug-free year my whole life was random and confusing and out of control. I could be perfectly normal then suddenly lose it. This happened not long after my crazy phone call with the MP.

I was sitting in my parents' garden; I was alone and about to eat lunch when my mood shifted. It was almost a physical change, as if a new version of reality had been inserted into my brain and someone pressed 'play'. The way things were placed on the table started to annoy me. Why was the butter always on the left-hand side of the table and not the right-hand side? I couldn't stop thinking about it. My frustration built until I exploded, grabbed the table and heaved it over. Everything smashed on the ground. I kicked the chair across the garden as hard as possible. I walked in circles yelling and screaming and kicking at nothing. Images flashed before my eyes, a shrilling sound screeched in my ears, the pressure in my head was excruciating.

Then I heard voices, like a radio somewhere in the distance. I knew this was all 'their' fault and was sick of them. The voices became clearer. I could hear someone telling me I was an idiot and full of shit. I couldn't stand it, so I ran inside, tore open all the boxes of painkillers I could find and washed the lot down with a mug filled to the brim with warm cheap white wine.

After half an hour I started to feel settled. The bottle of wine and the pills had numbed me and a perverse sense of pleasure started to creep in. Now I felt good about being mad. I grabbed another bottle of wine and kept drinking and chain-smoking cigarettes. I was mad and crazy and loving it and wanted more. I hit full party mode, then realised I was stuck in the middle of nowhere by myself and it really pissed me off. So I grabbed my diary:

I'm sitting here pumped full of alcohol and codeine, thinking, procrastinating. I've ended up in the living room of a deserted farmhouse, but all I think about is being in a coma. Everything sucks, everything is fucked. I want to get away. I want to get away. Because being here makes me crazy. I have so much energy, I want to live. I don't want to sit here staring at the same trees. There are no freaks here, not even straight people, only kangaroos, but they don't want to get stoned. What is the point of looking at kangaroos when they don't want to join the party? It doesn't make sense, why are they there? Where is my future, is it the drug path? Who knows?

Reading that entry really shocked me. The diary was supposed to have been a journal of my psychedelic adventures in the romantic hippie tradition, but for some reason I kept writing long after that journey derailed. Those entries brought back other memories of how I felt at that time, and illustrated what a confused and terrible state I was in.

WHAT HAPPENS DURING PSYCHOSIS

As I treated more clients with psychosis and remembered more about what I had been through, I saw that rather than being chaotic and random, psychotic episodes arise from a progression of organ imbalances. Psychosis is logical and predictable, including the voices and delusions. My clients weren't mad or showing symptoms of mental illness, they were suffering specific organ imbalances and deficiencies. In my post-drug depleted state my damaged liver was unable to keep inner energy flowing, so I couldn't make sense of my physical environment. When your chi becomes stagnant, this manifests as irritability. You resist your physical environment. Nothing looks or feels right. You can't perceive harmony because yin and yang are not in harmony with each other.

My drug-depleted kidneys were too weak to balance yin and yang so I felt I was losing my power. This makes you angry. My lungs were too deficient to control my anger, and I started blaming others for everything. My spleen couldn't digest what was going on. As my thoughts couldn't be moved, they began to loop. This developed into uncontrollable obsession. I was trapped. I couldn't move mentally or physically.

> Psychosis is logical and predictable, including the voices and delusions. My clients weren't mad or showing symptoms of mental illness, they were suffering specific organ imbalances and deficiencies.

When your spleen is too deficient to allow you to feel centred, you're not sure what is real and what isn't, and you don't know what to do about it. You're confused and not in flow with life. As the stagnation of the chi reaches a critical point, it threatens to separate body (yin) and mind (yang). If yin and yang

When your spleen is too deficient to allow you to feel centred, you're not sure what is real and what isn't, and you don't know what to do about it. You're confused and not in flow with life. As the stagnation of the chi reaches a critical point, it threatens to separate body (yin) and mind (yang). If yin and yang fully separate the outcome will be death.

● ● ● ● ● ● ● ●

fully separate the outcome will be death. To prevent this your liver increases the urge to advance and act (yang), to make sure the situation changes. This in turn creates heat and your anger intensifies.

The heat makes the looping thoughts and images come to life. They cannot be controlled anymore. They overwhelm you. Heat rises and expands as far as it can, to the ears. As the ears are a sophisticated receptor box, the heat changes their physiology. Now you are receiving more than one frequency. You can hear things you can't make sense of.

As your organs are seriously depleted this information is filtered through a deficient kidney (causing fear), a deficient spleen (causing confusion), and a depleted liver (causing anger). As nothing is resolved, the heat intensifies into fire and affects your heart.

Now your heart, the home of your mind, is on fire. As your mind is you, you panic. You have to escape the confusion, the images and the voices. You feel your anger increasing, giving you the energy to escape but also making the images and voices become more real. Your spleen is unable to digest all this, or transport you out of it, so you feel your life is now under serious threat. You need to take control, so you lash out and become violent.

After this your body eventually returns to balance. The fire has burned out what was left of your inner resources. You are depleted, exhausted and ashamed. You want to die; you sit there and cry. The tears (metal element) are the clouds which provide the rain. The rain builds the water element, the water nourishes the wood element and it makes the wood grow. Growth is yang. The yang slowly starts to build. But, because you have a depleted organ system you cannot balance the yang with the necessary yin, so the chi cannot flow. The pressure mounts, and the cycle starts again.

OBSESSIONS AND THE SPLEEN

The reason for my speed-obsessive behaviour seems clear to me now, but at the time I had no idea what was happening. People did all sorts of strange repetitive things. We knew it was speed-related but thought no more of it.

In traditional Chinese medicine this looping is associated with the spleen. If you have a healthy spleen you are able to resolve thoughts, ideas and actions instantly, but ongoing speed use damages this function. You can't resolve anything you are engaged in, physical or intellectually. 'Tweaking' is a term some of my clients use to describe this behaviour. I treated one young guy who had really long curly hair which his parents disapproved of. One night he decided he wanted to cut a little bit off to make a fringe. He was after a certain style that he had seen in a magazine. Once he started cutting, though, he got trapped in cutting. By the next morning he practically had a crew-cut. His parents were very impressed, thinking it was a sign that he was changing and becoming more responsible.

Obsessive behaviour increases in intensity the more drugs you take, due to their action on the spleen and other organs. In my day we were all careful to keep that kind of thing within the scene. I constantly monitored my emotions and corrected myself with the relevant mood-and mind-altering substances. Different occasions required different 'medications'. If I had a family function to attend, I would take a combination of drugs that could make me feel internally high but externally appear calm. I would always make sure my visits ended well before the drugs wore off and my behaviour deteriorated.

These management strategies were only effective up to a certain point, though. If you keep using speed, ice or other hard drugs, your actions become more extreme and much less entertaining to yourself and

> If you keep using speed, ice or other hard drugs, your actions become more extreme and much less entertaining to yourself and others, particularly when they keep happening long after you give the drugs away.

others, particularly when they keep happening long after you give the drugs away. Eventually you will collide with the external world and someone will stop you.

28 OVERCOMING PSYCHOSIS

The link between amphetamines (benzedrine) and psychosis has been recognised in the west since the 1930s. As amphetamine use increased dramatically after World War II, more cases emerged,[1] but the condition was still believed to be rare. By 1953 research from several different countries had identified only a small number of cases.[2] But with the current epidemic of recreational amphetamine and methamphetamine (speed) use, psychosis has become commonplace.

I believe that the incidence of psychosis is increasing because more people are taking drugs and are using much more powerful drugs such as crystal meth or ice (crystal methamphetamine hydrochloride), a powerful synthetic stimulant far more potent than other forms of amphetamine. Whereas speed has a purity of ten to twenty percent, ice is eighty percent pure. It is estimated that a quarter of regular ice users will experience psychosis.[3]

People have different ways of handling their psychosis. Kevin, a dope-dealer in his forties, had been using speed, cocaine and ice for twenty years. He lived in the country and had a large dope plantation hidden in the forest nearby. One night just before he dropped off to sleep, Kevin heard the faint sound of a helicopter. The noise grew louder as it flew closer. Then he heard cars pull up as well. There were people outside his windows speaking on walkie-talkies and a police radio crackled in the background. Kevin's heart started pounding as he realised that the police were surrounding his house to bust him for the drugs. He panicked and jumped out a side window to escape but there was no one out there.

A week later the same thing happened. Again Kevin ran outside in a panic and again there was no one there. As this kept happening, he finally worked out a plan. Once he heard the helicopter and the cars he would go to the toilet and flush it several times so the imaginary cops would think he had disposed of his drug stash. They would then leave and he could go back to sleep. He might have got that scenario under control, but as he kept using ice things intensified until one night he was arrested for running down a street nude and shouting abuse. He was taken to the emergency ward of a hospital where he was restrained and medicated.

Kevin had a really strong constitution, which is ideal for heavy drug users. He had been using hard drugs for decades, and had become used to the delusions, voices and uncomfortable states. He had learned how to differentiate between what was and was not real. But because he kept using drugs the yang imbalance eventually became too strong, and he ended up restrained in hospital. This is becoming much more common now with huge increases in the numbers of cases of psychosis admitted to hospital emergency wards. I have had several clients (speed and ice users) who were so convinced that people were after them that they called the police. The police would turn up to find the client there with a lot of drugs and nothing else.

BUGS ON THE SKIN

The symptoms of psychosis include delusions, paranoia, fear of persecution and visual and auditory hallucinations. I have also had a few clients who, after using ice, speed or cocaine, were convinced they had bugs crawling over or under their skin. One client, a heavy speed user, was so sure he had lice he went to a doctor, who sent him to a psychiatrist who told him he was psychotic and prescribed medication.

In traditional Chinese medicine this feeling of bugs on the skin is due to yang rising and heat in the blood. The chi flow is interrupted and alternates between rapid flow and stagnation. This manifests as prickles of heat under the skin, which feels like ants or insects biting. A lot of people these days have itchy skin. This is a milder form of the same imbalance. These conditions can be effectively treated with professionally prescribed Chinese raw herbs and acupuncture.

YANG SOCIETY

Our lifestyle is also contributing to the increase in psychosis, as we are becoming a more yang society with our information and communications-based culture. Our computers, mobile phones and high-tech gadgets are yang. The highly processed, high-sugar and high-fat foods we eat are an excess of yang. As a result obesity is increasing.

The 'tube' body shape of the new generation often has noticeable fat distribution around the middle and hips. In traditional Chinese medicine, this area is the girdle channel, which regulates the balance between the upward and downward flow of life energy. Fat in this section represents a massive stagnation or concentration of energy due to its interrupted downward flow. This indicates a drifting apart of body and mind. Energy accumulates in the upper body, so our shoulders hunch and the neck tightens, pushing the head forward. Energy then gets stuck at the back of the neck. This accounts for chronic headaches and irritability. Food does not sink, so bloating occurs. You don't feel grounded.

Increased yang needs to be matched by an increase in yin, through eating regular nutritious meals, exercising and developing the ability to sit with one thing at a time without becoming distracted. We have lost this skill. It is common for my clients to watch TV, listen to music, answer emails and phone calls, send text messages, get dressed and eat breakfast all at the same time. This behaviour is a precursor of disease.

All these factors predispose people to the development of psychosis. If you add powerful stimulant (yang) drugs to a manic lifestyle, or even prescribed antidepressants, antipsychotics or attention deficit disorder drugs, the separation between body and mind accelerates. The flow of energy is further inhibited. Once the energy accumulation reaches a critical mass it has to find release. Outbursts of violence are a way of releasing excess energy. People talk about 'going off their heads' on drugs. This is actually a good description of excess yang escaping. It is no coincidence that we now have a new symptom associated with psychosis—violence.

29 PSYCHOSIS AND VIOLENCE

Leanne, a small, articulate and attractive 23-year-old woman, was my first 'violent' psychosis case. She used ice daily although, like many of my clients, she had a permanent job where no one had any idea she was a drug user. Over the weekend she would binge, then go out to the clubs and bars. One night Leanne had been drinking and chatting with people when she noticed a woman across the room flirting with her boyfriend. She got really annoyed, raced over and started abusing the woman, who denied everything. Leanne lost her temper and started screaming at the woman and was evicted by security.

Later, she found out her boyfriend wasn't even in the club that night and she was really embarrassed and confused. The same thing happened a few more times. Each time she would find out her boyfriend hadn't been there. She eventually split up with the boyfriend, but it kept happening even though she was now single. One night it went too far and Leanne dragged a girl outside the club and started hitting her. When the police arrived, Leanne was so physically out of control it took three policemen to restrain her. She spent the rest of that night in a cell.

By the time she finished telling me this story Leanne had her head in her hands. She was really ashamed of what she had done. I asked her what she was like when she was a child, and she said she had been really shy and timid.

She was too selfconscious to speak out in public, and had been brought up to believe that her opinions didn't have any value. As a teenager she couldn't express her emotions and felt weak. The first time she tried speed it turned her into an assertive, confident and outgoing person, the way she had always wanted to be. When she discovered ice, the effect intensified a hundred times over and she never looked back.

Like many of my clients, Leanne's energy temporarily lifted when she talked about the way the drugs made her feel, but she instantly corrected this. She wished she had never touched any drug, as she was now on antipsychotic medication and 'damaged beyond repair'. This made her feel powerless, the very thing that had driven her to recreational drugs in the first place. So she was back where she was before, but disillusioned, depressed and ashamed as well.

I explained to Leanne that we had to identify and work with the positives of what she had been through. She couldn't think of any positives. I said that in my opinion the psychosis had brought forward issues about powerlessness, fear, weakness and the inability to control her life. Her delusions kept playing out the scenario of someone taking her boyfriend. As he represented her means of attaining happiness, these delusions were about someone stealing happiness from her. In her pre-drug days she would have let that happen, because she felt unworthy of happiness. But in her psychotic state the yang overrode that old conditioning and allowed her to boldly confront anyone preventing her from finding happiness.

If she had never taken the drugs and subsequently become violent, she would always have thought of herself as weak. Now she had been shown she was in fact a lethal weapon. Leaving aside the moral implications, she had held off three big burly cops for twenty minutes. The amount of energy available to her in those twenty minutes was mind-blowing. And what was more mind-blowing was that all that power had been unleashed from within her. The drugs may have instigated it, but it was her own power that had been drawn upon. I suggested she imagine making that energy work for her and imagine the freedom she could experience if she could tap into that power to improve herself.

Leanne was too astonished to speak at first, as it was such a reversal of the way she saw herself. Then she asked how she could draw upon this power. I told her that the energy she had unleashed during her psychotic episode was from her body and that strength is not about muscles, it is about energy and will. Strength comes from training the body and the mind. The next step for her would be to train in a martial art to make that power accessible. Martial arts are not about learning to bash people, they are about learning to deal with and overcome obstacles. You learn to use the momentum of universal forces, and once you have a glimpse of that, it makes an ice high look like nothing. Leanne's psychosis had magnified an important soul issue and given her a clear sense of how she could be. By the end of the session, she realised the therapeutic potential her psychosis held for her. She enrolled in a martial arts school and over time learned how to control and build her own energies.

> Leanne's psychosis had magnified an important soul issue and given her a clear sense of how she could be. By the end of the session, she realised the therapeutic potential her psychosis held for her. She enrolled in a martial arts school and over time learned how to control and build her own energies.

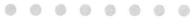

MEDICAL MANAGEMENT

Like many other drug users Leanne had been prescribed antipsychotic medication. However, in traditional Chinese medicine, uncontrollable violence and aggression result from excess yang. Each pharmaceutical drug that is administered exacerbates this problem by further depleting yin. I am not against medication. I also understand that when patients present in a hospital needing five people to restrain them, it is not really the environment in which to have a discussion about alternatives, or yin and yang. All drugs—recreational or pharmaceutical—have a role to play, but they are all temporary and I am looking at permanent solutions.

It is here that traditional Chinese medicine can contribute in both the critical and long-term phase. Acupuncture, if applied by a fully trained and experienced professional, can instantly remove excess yang. If hospital emergency wards employed trained acupuncturists who also had martial arts training, they could help deal with the immediate situation as well as advising on subsequent strategies for balancing yin and yang to prevent further psychotic incidents from occurring.

Just about everyone I see for psychosis has been medicated, but that is not enough. You can't heal psychosis by numbing it or suppressing it with medication, because the major issues underpinning this behaviour will still be there. These need to be tackled at the appropriate time, and lifestyle changes need to be implemented so that healing can take place.

You can't heal psychosis by numbing it or suppressing it with medication, because the major issues underpinning this behaviour will still be there. These need to be tackled at the appropriate time, and lifestyle changes need to be implemented so that healing can take place.

30 ICE, SEX AND VIOLENCE

Right after Leanne I saw another client, Sally, who had different issues with ice and violence. Sally had started smoking marijuana when she was thirteen, then discovered ecstasy when she was sixteen. She was a recreational user as it was occasional use and primarily connected with fun and socialising. When she turned twenty, one of her friends offered her ice. Like most people who think of trying hard drugs, she was hesitant at first, but then Sally decided to give it a go. It is usually a friend, or a friend of a friend, who introduces you to drugs. Their motives are generally not sinister. Drugs can make you feel so expansive and excited that you immediately want to share those feelings with other people.

It was the level of enthusiasm Sally's friend had for ice that convinced Sally to try it. When she did she had the most euphoric rush of her life and immediately wanted to do it again. Sally then raved about ice to her boyfriend, a dope-smoker who had never done hard drugs, not even ecstasy. He didn't want to try ice, but she was so passionate

> It is usually a friend, or a friend of a friend, who introduces you to drugs. Their motives are generally not sinister. Drugs can make you feel so expansive and excited that you immediately want to share those feelings with other people.

about it he was worried that if he didn't try it she would start moving in other circles. They smoked it in a pipe and he too was instantly captivated.

On ice their attraction to each other magnified a thousand times over. He and Sally had sex for eight hours. It was as if ice opened the door to endless sensual pleasure. Ice is a powerful yang drug, which means it has a major impact on the libido. It dramatically increases the desire for sex. On ice the discovery phase doesn't stop, so you can constantly discover new sexual pleasure, and this is a major attraction of the drug. A lot of my single male clients who use ice on the weekend, buy the drug and book sex-workers at the same time. Afterwards it is common for them to watch pornographic videos and masturbate for a few more hours.

> Ice is a powerful yang drug, which means it has a major impact on the libido. It dramatically increases the desire for sex. On ice the discovery phase doesn't stop, so you can constantly discover new sexual pleasure, and this is a major attraction of the drug.

Ice and hours of incredible sex became a regular weekend event for Sally and her boyfriend. They wanted to discover more and more intense forms of pleasure, so they increased the amount of ice they were using, until they were doing four continuous days of ice and sex. They were also bonding on a level they couldn't have imagined before, and thought ice had turned their relationship into pure bliss.

After a few months of this, Sally noticed a shift in herself. On the third day of their four-day sessions, instead of feeling a wild attraction to her boyfriend, he repelled her. She didn't want him to touch her. Using more ice exacerbated this feeling, so she would take dozens of sleeping pills and tranquillisers in order to sleep, breaking the cycle and creating a new starting point. Her boyfriend didn't want to stop, or to sleep. He was hooked on the yang and needed to keep going. He started going on five-day benders. Meanwhile they turned from exploring their attraction to each other and why they loved each other, to exploring the negative side of their relationship.

They became obsessed with what didn't work. Everything each of them did was interpreted by the other as a sign of opposition. They could no longer have a normal conversation, and the tension became unbearable. Sally started going out of her way to aggravate her boyfriend, and finally she provoked him to the point where he hit her. He had never been violent before but once it started, the violence escalated. He would hold knives to her throat, he raped her and one day dislocated her jaw. They became trapped in a cycle of violence. Sally began to feel afraid of him but didn't want to leave because they were so tightly bonded.

The ice had shown them incredible bliss, but it had also taken them way beyond the boundaries of emotional safety. It stripped away all the social niceties and they entered a world of primal emotions, rage, obsession and violence. Eventually the fights became so loud and out of control that the police were called. A restraining order was placed on the boyfriend and they could no longer see each other.

After this the boyfriend stopped using ice, but Sally couldn't let it go. She didn't want to go back to a normal life, she now needed the excess stimulation, excitement and intensity. She was drawn to the underworld, to drug-fuelled orgies, dealers and sex work. Although this world was unpredictable and dangerous, it also seemed glamorous.

Her family were worried about her new lifestyle. Her father told her she was an addict and had to give up, but if she stopped using ice she felt empty, trapped and alone. For Sally the issue wasn't just the drugs. If we focused purely on taking the ice out of the equation, her life would be bland. She needed to look at the bigger picture, at her psychosis. The way she described her year on ice revealed a highly inquisitive mind. Sally gave me an in-depth interpretation of all her actions on the drugs. It was as if she was actively participating in all the madness, while mentally recording every detail. I had the impression that instead of doing drugs she was undertaking empirical research.

HEALING

I believe some people incarnate into this world to go through certain experiences, so that they can then contribute to the evolution of healing modalities.

Quite a few of my clients fit into this category. I saw Sally as part of this group. The instant I mentioned it her eyes lit up. It made sense to her. I said if that was the case, she had done her practical and now it was time for the theory. She had to study then draw on her own experiences and those of her friends going through various drug-induced psychoses to develop a new treatment model for psychosis.

In our society any form of mental imbalance still tends to be shut away or suppressed with medication, but this doesn't heal the person. The next frontier in therapy is to *understand* mental imbalances from fresh perspectives and find new ways of working with these states. The wave of post-drug psychosis is going to force this to happen, and the most innovative solutions may well come from those who have both experiential and academic knowledge.

EXTREME BEHAVIOURS

Drug use is often connected with excessive behaviours that people are embarrassed about or ashamed of afterwards. Many are associated with sex. Sally was embarrassed about the orgies and all the people she had sex with while on drugs, and about selling herself for sex, but the ancient Chinese philosophers say that to help others you need worldly experience and drug users certainly have this. Rather than hiding your past, do something wonderful with it.

Many clients came to me feeling confused, ashamed or guilty about their obsessions, delusions and activities on drugs, but all those behaviours have arisen from various organ imbalances and were beyond the control of the person. However, they can offer valuable insight into your inner world. If we change the way we think about and treat psychosis, it could be a huge opportunity for growth.

PART VII:
A NEW TAKE ON PSYCHOSIS

31 SEEING PSYCHOSIS DIFFERENTLY

It was all very well to make grand claims about psychosis, but it wasn't until a meeting with the director of a drug rehab centre that I clarified my ideas on what was possible. He was interested in my 'working with drugs' approach. When we sat in his office I spoke enthusiastically about my program, and the power of traditional Chinese medicine, supplements, meditation and martial arts.

After about an hour he casually asked if I'd like to meet some of his clients. I followed him into an adjoining room. A ring of chairs faced me. A dozen really heavy-looking guys in jeans, T-shirts and caps pulled low were sitting staring at me. Most were aged between forty and fifty. They were long-term hardcore ex-addicts who had done time in jail and on the streets. I was right back in the drug world I had run away from as a youth worker and it looked as if nothing had changed.

The director must have planned the meeting but the guys had no idea who I was, and little interest in finding out. The talks I usually gave were based on my belief that drug experiences ultimately lead to self-realisation and spirituality, but these people had had such bad experiences, they no longer even believed in good.

When the director asked me to introduce myself, I realised I was on my own. It looked as if I'd walked into a twelve-step meeting. I wondered whether

I was expected to say I was an addict and alcoholic there to 'share', or whether I should present myself as someone who was going to help. I started talking about what I did, beginning with the present as an acupuncturist and winding back to my past as a speed addict and alcoholic, but no one was really engaged until I stated that addiction was not a disease and that if you are a drug user, simply giving up drugs is not the solution. If you have taken drugs they have opened doors and your responsibility is to walk through them. Now they were paying attention.

BRINGING THE BODY UP

I said there was a whole lot more going on with drugs than most people realise, and that humans are like a radio or TV, capable of receiving a huge range of frequencies. Most of us tend to be tuned into only one station, or commonly perceived reality. However, after drug use or other factors, you can pick up other stations. I talked about Dr Rick Strassman's work with the drug DMT. So many of his subjects had taken DMT and had contact with beings that he stopped passing off these experiences as hallucinations and started considering that those experiences were exactly what they seemed to be.[1] This led him to explore the idea of DMT allowing access to parallel universes, or planes of existence in dark matter. He proposed that there are different levels of reality present all the time, but they usually remain inaccessible to us. For some people the increased receptivity they attained while using drugs remains after they stop. The mind goes onto auto-scroll and a jumble of information streams through. It might be from somewhere forward in time, or from other planes of existence, or it may be from several realities at once. It is all real but incomprehensible. You know stuff, but you can't make any sense of it. You are diagnosed as psychotic, then medicated to shut off those other channels.

Everyone had shifted forward in their seats. One of the guys pushed his cap back and said he had used several grams of speed a day for years and was mentally fucked-up. He had heard voices and believed everyone was after him, from the government and the police to people in the street. He thought that there were microphones and cameras in every electronic device in his apartment. He took everything apart, from hairdryers to toasters.

Then the guy beside him said he too was psychotic and heard voices. For years he thought everyone was carrying stun guns to knock him out and take him away, so he constantly attacked people. He ended up in and out of jail and psych wards. Others started telling their stories. They had all been psychotic.

Energy started firing through me. I had seen far too many passionate and creative people who had taken drugs and as a result unwittingly opened themselves up to other frequencies, then been told they were mentally ill. The medication took away the symptoms, but also their reason to live. Their lives had become nothing, and their eyes were defeated. Facing a room full of these guys all saying the same thing at once brought home how destructive it was to write people off, and medicate, suppress and condemn them.

These guys were not permanently mentally ill. Their organs were depleted from the drugs, alcohol, pain and junk food. I told them drugs initially make the world look fantastic because they enhance the function of every organ. Speed or ice

For some people the increased receptivity they attained while using drugs remains after they stop. The mind goes onto auto-scroll and a jumble of information streams through. It might be from somewhere forward in time, or from other planes of existence, or it may be from several realities at once. It is all real but incomprehensible. You know stuff, but you can't make any sense of it. You are diagnosed as psychotic, then medicated to shut off those other channels.

I had seen far too many passionate and creative people who had taken drugs and as a result unwittingly opened themselves up to other frequencies, then been told they were mentally ill. The medication took away the symptoms, but also their reason to live.

pump up the function of the kidneys, which are responsible for mental and physical strength. That is why you feel like Mr Universe and can have sex for hours on end. Everyone nodded—they all knew that feeling. For the drugs to create that effect, they harm the kidneys so that eventually you get fear instead of willpower and strength. Add in the damaged spleen, you get confusion. Add in the damaged liver and anger joins the mix.

No wonder you think the cops, aliens or passers-by are after you. You feel you are in danger, so to survive you attack. What they needed to do was upgrade their bodies. Medication is about bringing the mind down, but they could also focus on bringing the body up. This is the answer to psychosis. You don't bring the mind down, you bring the body up. You catch up to your mind, you make it work for you. We are here to evolve and this is what evolution is about.

> This is the answer to psychosis. You don't bring the mind down, you bring the body up. You catch up to your mind, you make it work for you. We are here to evolve and this is what evolution is about.

● ● ● ● ● ● ● ●

The guy who had been in jail for violence asked how to make his screwed-up mind work for him. I told him he could develop his enhanced receptivity into intuition, then work as a counsellor or therapist helping others. When people came to him, he would be able to instantly sense what needed to be corrected. His face changed for an instant. His eyes lit up. This was something that inspired him, but a second later it was gone. The old programming had shut it down. He was a huge, dangerous-looking guy, with arms covered in tattoos. I said, 'Look at you. Your past is written all over you. Can you imagine if you recaptured everything you had on drugs, what a powerhouse of attraction and inspiration you would be to other drug users? You would be walking charisma. You wouldn't need fancy academic words or theories, because your presence would say it all. The future needs people like you, drug warriors who inspire by example.'

BECOMING A DRUG WARRIOR

Part of being a drug warrior means facing and resolving your past. He cut in, saying, 'Mate, no one could resolve my past. I had to live on the streets from when I was nine. I had to fight just to stay alive. I thought everyone was after me and started bashing people just because they looked at me wrong.' He paused for a moment, then added, 'But I didn't want to be like that.' I told him that no one does. He probably had such imbalances he was simply unable to control himself. What was missing for him was the yin. I had a client who was in fights every day. When he discovered tai-chi, everything changed. Within weeks his aggression had noticeably lessened, because the tai-chi gave him 'space' and techniques to observe himself before reacting.

I explained that if he took up a practice such as that, then worked with his increased receptivity, it meant he would not be trapped in one version of reality any more. He could look at everything from a bigger perspective. He could even get outside all of the emotionality of the pain and see why he was born in that environment. They say we all choose to reincarnate in a specific family for a specific reason. Instead of just being the victim and the loser, he could get the big picture of how he was involved. Anger in itself is without value. It is there to motivate you to create change. It gives you the focus and power to concentrate on your pain and resolve it. You need to be able to look at your anger and understand its true nature.

We talked more about how to upgrade the body, and how martial arts bring the body up to the speed of the mind. Some martial artists are so quick that in order for all their moves to be seen, they have to be filmed, then the footage has to be slowed down when screened. I showed them some of the tai-chi moves I worked with to unify my body and mind. We also discussed the specific weight-training programs to correct the imbalances that lead to psychosis, and what muscle groups to target.

Our meeting became an incredibly charged experience. Towards the end, I talked about turning pain into love. That last part came out spontaneously. This was not an environment in which I would usually introduce such an idea.

Expressing love is difficult for anyone, but particularly so if you have come from a background of constant pain and abuse. But because I had taken them rationally through all the dark and crazy territory first, they felt comfortable enough to entertain this idea. If I had opened with such a concept it would have been a different story.

Without real insight into the terrible pain and confusion many ex-users battle daily, it is almost impossible to give them a vision of life beyond those states. It is within the destruction that the seeds of creation lie. When you understand this, everything is possible.

32 TURNING PAIN INTO LOVE

How do you turn pain into love? There are long traditions of using suffering as a means of learning and self-transformation in many cultures. In the west, this approach of turning pain into love was replaced with modern psychiatry, which identifies diseases of the mind and prescribes medication, just as doctors identify the diseases of the body and prescribe medication. So people who have been through psychosis do not have the opportunity to gain any insight from their experiences. Psychosis can be a gift as it enables us to consciously access the subconscious. The thoughts or actions that emerge are significant. Basically, our delusions or obsessions can be a powerful diagnostic tool, as what surfaces in delusional states is not totally random but holds a wealth of information about the person.

Psychosis can be a gift as it enables us to consciously access the subconscious. The thoughts or actions that emerge are significant. Basically our delusions or obsessions can be a powerful diagnostic tool, as what surfaces in delusional states is not totally random. It holds a wealth of information about the person.

This does need to be interpreted correctly and this is not a straightforward process. Because vast amounts of information are accessible, the mind employs complex visual imagery to communicate it. This information is coded, as in your dreams, which seem logical while you are dreaming but make no sense when you wake up. A major branch of therapy is based on dream interpretation. This is the direction to take in working with some psychoses. My training in pulse diagnosis is also useful as I not only observe the physical aspects of the pulses; I've learned to work with and interpret symbolic language as well. When you put these skills together you get a key to decode psychotic episodes.

When people are in psychotic states, they are usually told their version of reality is incorrect. They are put under tremendous pressure to conform to the commonly perceived version of reality. This exacerbates the problem. If you are psychotic you often no longer have the ability to move. Forcing someone in that state to shift back to 'normal' reality can create a negative reaction. This was noted as early as the mid-twentieth century by such renowned psychiatrists as RD Laing. Laing proposed new ways of looking at mental imbalances. He considered that in psychotic states people were attempting to communicate serious concerns, often in situations where this was not possible or not permitted. He interacted with these patients on the basis that their delusions represented valid descriptions of reality rather than symptoms of an underlying disorder.[1]

PSYCHOSIS AS EVOLUTIONARY ADVANTAGE

Working *with* psychosis, rather than against it, enables a more positive outcome. More contemporary research might lead us further down that road. In new evolutionary psychiatry, it has been suggested that some mental disorders are not even pathologies but strategies that make evolutionary sense. From this perspective there could be evolutionary advantages in psychosis. When you are in a psychotic state you are disconnected from normal reality, but also from social pressures. This could be advantageous at times because we are such a highly social species.[2]

My psychological disturbances certainly intensified under social pressure. After my family joined me in Australia I became seriously delusional and it was no coincidence. At the time I was lucky to be living in a hippie commune where it was acceptable to have your own version of reality, so I could feel relatively safe within my madness. As a result, I was slowly starting to heal. When they arrived I went back to speed and over the edge. The day before they were due, I was sitting in a hippie restaurant very drunk and stoned. It was my favourite place. There was no judgement, no hierarchy, no expectations. I had the horrifying realisation that within twenty-four hours my family were going to walk back into my life with their straight eyes, straight values, straight expectations and judgements. My safety structure collapsed around me. Panic and fear closed my throat.

The truth was, I didn't want to see my family. I just wanted to be left alone for a very, very long time, to gain the psychological stability I needed to deal with them on my own terms. But I had been brought up to believe that family was important. My social conditioning was so deeply ingrained that I couldn't say I didn't want to see them. By the time they arrived I was so frightened I was totally manic. We had arranged to meet in that same cafe. It was a terrible evening. People came over to chat but I was incapable of interacting with them and my relatives at the same time. The two versions of reality clashed so badly there was no common ground between them. It was only then that I understood that I had been temporarily free, and that freedom was essential for my survival.

PARANOID DELUSIONS

Initially everyone seemed pleased to see me so tanned and healthy, as I had left Germany a pale, skeletal speed addict. As soon as I stopped using speed I started to put on weight. As speed is a yang drug, it takes away your hunger and accelerates your metabolism. The body burns everything up. After speed everything slows down again. Speed also damages the function of the spleen and stomach, contributing to weight gain and fluid retention.

After the novelty of my appearance wore off, it didn't take long for the chains to tighten. I ended up agreeing to leave the commune and move in with my family. We had to go on a four-day car trip together to get to their new property. At that stage I was topping up with pills every couple of hours just to keep myself in control. I couldn't do this in front of them so I bought bottles of cough mixture, tipped some out, then added vast amounts of ground-up painkillers. I changed the label on one bottle to make it look like it had come from a herbal shop so I could take it without revealing my dependency. I also packed six casks of wine, saying I'd got them on special. This denial and secrecy increased the pressure. I felt suffocated and smothered as I had when I was a small child. Moving back in with the family meant I was faced with those repressive forces again. Not long after, my paranoid delusional behaviour intensified.

The first serious episode happened at dinner time. Family meals were always highly stressful and one particular night I was more uptight than usual. Electricity crackled around me and I could hear sounds I couldn't identify. Then a loud, authoritative knock at the door startled me. Someone was after me. I asked my mother to open the door, as I didn't want 'them' to know I was there. Everyone looked at each other, then at me. No one had heard a knock. My anxiety increased. I couldn't understand why they didn't believe me and if no one opened the door, whoever was there might storm it. However, if I opened the door and pretended I didn't know why 'they' were there, hopefully 'they' would go away.

So, I ran and opened the door, but there was no one there. When I got back to the table no one said anything. They resumed their meals and conversations, but the atmosphere was painful. I let it go as long as I could before saying, 'They must still be here.' Someone tried to tell me no one had knocked, but I couldn't concentrate. A car had approached the house. 'They' were outside. I ran to the door, but again there was no one there. By now I was highly agitated and I ended up searching the grounds and the woods nearby.

WHO ARE THEY AND WHY ARE THEY AFTER ME?

Believing people are pursuing you is common in psychosis. I didn't know who 'they' were but wasn't surprised they were after me. Of course people had genuinely been after me for a long time. In Germany, due to my illicit activities, the police were always watching me and photographing me, and they had tried to bust me several times. Then, when my friends and I occupied an abandoned building as part of the squatter movement, it was surrounded by armies of police, which was very frightening.

I was a deserter from national service, so the military were after me too. Then there were repeated runs across borders while smuggling. I had a lot of unresolved and suppressed fear stored in my body and mind, which may have contributed to persecutory delusions. On top of that my organs were so depleted from the drugs, they were generating constant fear rather than willpower and strength.

I also had the feeling that my family were 'after me' to be part of something I didn't want. My persecutory delusions were also presenting this information to me in a symbolic manner. I didn't understand that at the time, though. My response was to drink even more to dampen the awful frantic energy in my head and stop my mind rambling off. I had casks of wine stashed all over the property so I could top myself up throughout the day and then, at meal times, go through the elaborate pretence of opening a bottle of wine, offering it around, and only having a glass or two myself. I was revelling in the idea that they would think I was normal like them, when in fact I had been drunk for hours.

PROPHET SYNDROME

The increased alcohol seemed to suppress the persecutory aspect of my paranoia, or maybe the pressure was just too much. I shifted from believing that I was being persecuted to thinking I had been chosen. From then on everything and everyone I came across were messengers informing me of my destiny.

One day on the property I found a newborn lamb whose mother must have died. As far as I was concerned it was a sign I was to be a shepherd, a leader of lost souls. The lamb had to be by my side as a symbol of my role. A few days later someone told me it was a goat. I stuck to the plan anyway, named it Schroeder, and it became my constant companion.

Schroeder and I were to travel the country, spreading wisdom in exchange for money and food. I made myself a wooden staff and shoulder bag, and sewed some colourful long robes then set out with Schroeder to save the world. We never made it past the local shopping centre, where people stared, pointed and laughed. I thought this was because they recognised my higher calling. I always made sure I walked in a regal manner, as befitted my special status. As far as my family were concerned, I was a source of embarrassment and annoyance. Looking back, my 'prophet syndrome' was connected with an imbalance in the fire element. I was no longer able to organise my ideas into logical, communicable language, a function of this element. Fire is also associated with our spirit. When fire is out of control, your reality is filtered by your spiritual beliefs and background. That's why many alcoholics in delirium suddenly think they are Jesus.

> The increased alcohol seemed to suppress the persecutory aspect of my paranoia, or maybe the pressure was just too much. I shifted from believing that I was being persecuted to thinking I had been chosen.

● ● ● ● ● ● ● ●

> Looking back, my 'prophet syndrome' was connected with an imbalance in the fire element. I was no longer able to organise my ideas into logical, communicable language, a function of this element. Fire is also associated with our spirit. When fire is out of control, your reality is filtered by your spiritual beliefs and background. That's why many alcoholics in delirium suddenly think they are Jesus.

● ● ● ● ● ● ● ●

As I was always interested in the idea of the travelling warrior/monk, this may have been where my own messianic vision originated.

In retrospect I think the idea that psychosis could have evolutionary advantages makes sense, because my messianic phase was also a survival tactic. Commonly perceived reality was not working for me. I felt under threat from the society I was in, so I retreated into a different version of reality. Unlike the persecutory delusions, I lived the messiah delusion. As it turned out, it was a much better place to be. I was happier during that period of my life, because I felt I had a purpose.

33 MARIJUANA, PSYCHOSIS AND DELUSIONS

In mainstream medicine my belief that I had been chosen would probably have been described as a grandiose delusion. Alex was my first client to report to me with this symptom.

He was supposedly psychotic, and grandiose delusions were part of this. Alex had smoked marijuana regularly since he was seventeen, and was now twenty. He had started to have manic episodes. He would be up for days furiously scribbling down ideas without following anything through. He talked incessantly to his parents and anyone else he met about everything he was going to do. He believed he could become rich overnight, because he knew what people wanted. His straight, hardworking parents thought he needed a kick in the arse to remind him what reality was.

After reading a number of articles about marijuana and psychosis, they decided Alex must have marijuana-induced psychosis. Marijuana has been getting a lot of bad press. Its use in adolescence has now been associated with mental disorders and schizophrenia, amongst other things.[1] I have not had a case where I could make this direct connection, but there have been significant changes in the marijuana being consumed, and the pattern of use, that might create imbalances in the organs that would generate psychotic symptoms.

Hydroponic marijuana is much more potent than the old 'bush weed' and is often saturated with toxic chemicals. From the traditional Chinese medicine perspective, marijuana is connected with the liver and wood element. It sets up an interaction between wood (ideas) and fire (excitement). Weak dope is like green wood that is hard to burn. Strong dope is like fast-burning wood that makes a nice big bright fire. As hydroponic marijuana is not grown in soil it does not have the grounding provided by the earth element (the yin), so there is no inhibition in the burning. Using hydroponic marijuana is like feeding a fire with petrol-saturated wood.

For the user this means a rush of ideas and excitement, and no inhibition. Many people who smoke a lot of hydroponic dope are overwhelmed with excitement and ideas. However, if they are yin depleted, water or kidney depleted, or have a weak constitution, the excess of ideas and excitement can run out of control. This can set the ground for the panic and delusions that fit the description of psychosis. In my experience, in many marijuana psychosis cases, either hard drugs were also involved or the person's lifestyle created such serious imbalances that the marijuana was the *trigger* for the psychosis, but was not the *cause* of it.

Weak dope is like green wood that is hard to burn. Strong dope is like fast-burning wood that makes a nice big bright fire. As hydroponic marijuana is not grown in soil it does not have the grounding provided by the earth element (the yin), so there is no inhibition in the burning. Using hydroponic marijuana is like feeding a fire with petrol-saturated wood.

● ● ● ● ● ● ● ●

Many people who smoke a lot of hydroponic dope are overwhelmed with excitement and ideas. However, if they are yin depleted, water or kidney depleted, or have a weak constitution, the excess of ideas and excitement can run out of control. This can set the ground for the panic and delusions that fit the description of psychosis.

● ● ● ● ● ● ● ●

Alex was told by his doctor to stop using marijuana as it was contributing to his behaviour, and he was given antipsychotic medication instead. His manic episodes went, but so too did his visions, ideas and creativity, and he became depressed and suicidal. His doctor added antidepressants to his medications, but Alex didn't feel better so he stopped taking all the medication and started smoking marijuana again. It seemed to kick him out of the depression.

Alex was confused. He felt worse on medication and better on marijuana, yet the marijuana was supposed to be the root of his problem. I explained that in his manic states his system was getting faster and faster, so he was getting inundated with ideas he couldn't process. This was making life uncomfortable for him as well as for his family. The medication took the 'fire' out of the visions, dampened the flow of ideas and gave him a chance to recover. But from what he was telling me, he needed these visions, otherwise he felt depressed and empty.

When we talked about his childhood he said that from day one he had hated school as it was boring, so he doodled on paper, looked out the window or imagined he was somewhere else. He was then diagnosed with attention deficit disorder (ADD) and put on amphetamine-based medication for the rest of his school days. When I asked about his diet he said as a child he rarely had breakfast, but would have a can of soft drink on his way to school. His mother sometimes made him sandwiches for lunch, but usually he would get chips and soft drink from the school canteen instead. After school he would snack on sweets and play computer games. When his parents got home at night they were stressed and exhausted, so they would often eat frozen meals or take-aways in front of the TV. This lifestyle had continued after he finished school.

THE QUICK FIX

I hear this story all the time, and each time it strikes a blow to my heart. In his childhood Alex had the lifestyle of a drug user—junk food and amphetamines. I was nineteen by the time I was doing that, and it was my choice. I knew drugs were bad for me. At least I'd had a chance to build some organ strength in my youth. Living like this from the age of five or six is devastating for the organs.

It is no wonder so many young people display psychotic symptoms so early in life. Then antidepressants or antipsychotic medications are prescribed, and the medication cycle continues. We have Prozac to thank for this. It was so heavily marketed to treat clinical depression that doctors began to diagnose depression in everyone. This led to the professional and public misconception that emotional disorders result from chemical imbalances in the brain and can be fixed with a pill. This became the model for the subsequent epidemic of children's psychiatric disorders and prescriptions of stimulant drugs for children who were dreamy, forgetful or simply disinterested in school.[2]

These days it is unusual for me to treat a young person who has not been on antidepressants or ADD drugs. I remember asking one young client if he had ever taken antidepressants and he said, 'No, apart from the usual years during high school that everybody does.' With this overmedication of children it should be no surprise that the next generation are turning to illicit drugs. It is not just about being born into a mind-set where so many people are using drugs. They have to use drugs because their organs are so depleted from their lifestyle

> In his childhood Alex had the lifestyle of a drug user—junk food and amphetamines. I was nineteen by the time I was doing that, and it was my choice. I knew drugs were bad for me. At least I'd had a chance to build some organ strength in my youth. Living like this from the age of five or six is devastating for the organs.

● ● ● ● ● ● ● ●

> These days it is unusual for me to treat a young person who has not been on antidepressants or ADD drugs. I remember asking one young client if he had ever taken antidepressants and he said, 'No, apart from the usual years during high school that everybody does.'

● ● ● ● ● ● ● ●

and medications that they need powerful drugs to fire up the organs with enough energy to get a sense of wellbeing. Also, if you spend your childhood or adolescence medicated, it is not a great leap to continue to chemically alter your mood.

Alex told me he had three or four pipes in the afternoon or evening. I was taken aback as this is not heavy use by current standards. I have clients who smoke ten or twenty times that each day. When he smoked dope Alex was able to sit with one idea rather than flying from one thing to another. I explained that marijuana allowed him to experience the creative flow again, but not in a manic way as it also provided 'space' (yin). This was probably why he thought it lifted his depression.

According to my diagnostics, marijuana wasn't the problem. Everything else was the problem—the medications he had been put on as a child, being brought up in a culture in which children have soft drinks and sugar for breakfast and don't ever eat a decent meal, and growing up in a society that does not provide what young people yearn for.

Then we discussed Alex's manic episodes. I explained that in traditional Chinese medicine any form of manic disorder is yang in nature. The root cause in his case was an organ imbalance and a deficiency of yin due to his lifestyle. If he wanted to benefit from his ideas he had to build his yin, which would create balance and allow him to carry out his ideas rather than just talk about them. Basically, each time he talked about his ideas it was too 'out there' (yang), so whoever he was speaking to would automatically correct him, to provide the missing yin. Whenever he spoke to his parents about the things he wanted to do, they told him that his ideas were unrealistic, and that if he wanted to get anywhere, he had to work hard at a normal job like everyone else. They were reacting to his imbalances.

GRAND VISION POTENTIAL

The problem was that Alex needed to talk about his visions to help him feel good about himself. The only way to break the cycle would be to not talk about his ideas but *become* them. If he focused on developing yin qualities, this would happen. Happiness and success are for those who follow the path of yin and yang.

I asked Alex for more details about his ideas and projects. One big idea after another tumbled out of his mouth. He was going to make movies, produce interactive games, invent new technologies and much, much more. Within minutes he produced half a dozen professional sketches illustrating a range of products and concepts. He definitely had his finger on the pulse and I told him so. He looked shocked. He said that when he mentioned his ideas people usually told him to shut up. I explained that if you can imagine it, you can do it. Maybe back in pre-human days some monkey talked about how he was going to be a human and live in cities and drive cars and fly to the moon. The other monkeys told him he was crazy, but some monkeys did in fact go on to that! We are in a universe of limitless potential.

Alex wasn't delusional, he had 'grand vision potential'. We can all have brilliant ideas and grand visions, but it is the ability to *implement* those ideas that makes them beneficial. To implement his ideas Alex needed to build yin by adopting a totally different lifestyle. I suggested he start by making little changes, like having regular acupuncture to control his hyper states, and getting rhythm and routine into his life. This builds yin. Eventually it would give him the power to control himself, so others wouldn't need to control him by putting him down verbally or with medication.

Changing the way you live is a really simple solution but it often takes people a very long time to grasp it. Most of us are just not brought up to understand how to live. Every patient I have treated for varying symptoms of psychosis, whether it was connected with drug use or not, lacked the physical grounding to be able to benefit from the speed of their mind and their ideas and visions. Once they made lifestyle changes, dramatic and constant improvements occurred.

> Changing the way you live is a really simple solution but it often takes people a very long time to grasp it. Most of us are just not brought up to understand how to live.

34 PSYCHOSIS AND PERSONAL GROWTH

The way Alex's family reacted to him made me realise how much I must have annoyed my family, who constantly criticised my behaviour hoping it would make me stop, as in their eyes I was doing something wrong. Stanislav Grof believed many of the conditions now considered psychoses are actually difficult stages of a radical personality transformation and spiritual opening.

> Stanislav Grof believed many of the conditions now considered psychoses are actually difficult stages of a radical personality transformation and spiritual opening. Correctly understood and supported, he thought these crises could lead to healing and the evolution of consciousness.

Correctly understood and supported, he thought these crises could lead to healing and the evolution of consciousness.[1] He probably wasn't referring to post-drug psychosis, but his ideas are still applicable.

I started wondering whether my psychosis was not only a survival strategy, but also held the potential for a major personal transformation. During my psychosis I was convinced that I had been chosen for something. A sign would show me my path. I didn't know when this would occur, but one day when my goat Schroeder and I were out walking, an overwhelmingly sacred feeling surged through me. It was so intensely joyous that tears poured down my face and I fell to my knees and looked up to heaven. I knew this was the sign I had been waiting for. I vowed to commit to the path of good, and that from then on all my life would be devoted to this.

REAL DELUSIONS

This event did feel real to me at the time, but I would never have dared think about it in terms of personal transformation as terms like 'mentally ill' and 'mad' had become attached to me. I now believe I went through my messianic stage because there was something in me that needed urgent attention. The delusions of persecution may have been connected with my issues of powerlessness and not living in accord with my true nature. I didn't get the message, so it was delivered in another way with the messiah trip. Looking back I think the message was about my life purpose.

As a child I was fascinated by religion and the supernatural but was repeatedly told there was no God, no life after death and so on, which always deeply hurt me. Drugs enabled me to connect with my longing for things of the spirit. My delusional, psychotic and obsessive actions were expressing a suppressed desire to be on a spiritual path.

When I emerged from my 'prophet' period, I knew I had created a lot of unpleasant and uncomfortable situations, so I moved to another town and tried to be as normal as possible. I buried my past. With it I also buried the unresolved seeds of the psychosis. This was why, years later, I worried that each psychotic patient I treated would release something within me, but it never happened. Even when I was at the rehab centre speaking to that group of serious psychosis cases it was an inspirational event.

Still, the idea that something was going to 'come out' kept plaguing me. When I thought back to the last time it had happened, it was when I had been invited to lunch with a German couple, Inga and Dirk, who had attended several of my talks and seminars. They seemed interesting; Dirk was a music producer, and I was keen to hear the latest news from the German music scene. Little did

I know that Dirk had been an ice addict, had become psychotic and then been on heavy-duty medication for years. My talks had inspired him to give up the medication, but he misunderstood the message of the workshops—change your foundations first and reduce the medication later under medical supervision. Dirk didn't improve his diet, get therapy, take supplements or Chinese herbs, or get into an exercise routine, so without the medication his behaviour quickly became erratic. He would get up at 3 am and wander around outside, and was constantly receiving messages that he was spiritually enlightened.

Inga recognised the signs and had set up the lunch hoping I would be able to convince him of his state and need for medication. I had no idea about this until, as soon as I arrived, Inga excused herself. Suddenly understanding what she had done, Dirk thought I had tricked him too. I realised I would have to play a therapeutic role.

I mentioned that I wouldn't give up medication without major lifestyle changes first, such as the daily exercise and everything else outlined in my workshops. Dirk wasn't interested. He stared at me intently and immediately told me that I was far too rigid and that I needed to be spontaneous to be on the spiritual path.

I had been doing my daily exercise, weights and tai-chi for years and the entire time I'd had to defend my practice to everyone from spiritual leaders to friends. People were constantly telling me I didn't need to be physically fit to be spiritual and that I was too obsessive about my practice. Even though I knew my program worked, I wasn't expecting this comment from Dirk and a flicker of insecurity crossed my mind.

Dirk was in such a heightened state he could sense my doubt, so he didn't see the point in taking any advice from me. I knew where Dirk was psychologically, though, because I had been there. Sitting with him I suddenly remembered an incident from my past. After I had moved back in with my family and started using speed again, I was telling my mother that on LSD you get information from a higher realm that you are expected to follow up on. I explained that I had been given the message that two of my relatives were under destructive influences and I had to correct this to protect the rest of the family. My mother thought I was crazy, which made me more determined to make her understand.

I felt uncomfortable thinking about what I had said and done that day but that memory came up for a reason, so I couldn't ignore it. In a psychotic state you may get specific insights into other people, but often these are about an issue you need to deal with. The problem is you are so imbalanced you cannot see this. My relatives were not under bad influences. What I was saying at the time wasn't about them, it was about me. Perhaps it was a call to heal myself, but my organs were so depleted that all incoming information took on a sinister aspect, and I projected my own imbalances onto others. Dirk was doing this too.

Psychosis presents us with an opportunity for self-development. It should not be permanently suppressed by medication, because that is spiritually wasteful. This sense of wasted opportunity frustrated me when I was speaking to the rehab group. They had been programmed to see themselves as diseased, mentally ill or having anger problems. What they needed was a post-psychosis lifestyle program to rebuild their health, then counselling to interpret the symbolic messages inherent in their psychotic activities. As Dirk illustrated at our lunch, you might know things when you are psychotic but it is not until you understand them in relation to yourself that you can make them useful.

35 PROCESSING PSYCHOSIS

After Alex, my first grandiose delusion client, I started treating people who, like me, had used drugs, become psychotic and recovered, but had the sense that some residue of the psychosis was still there, and that something could trigger it again. Working with them led me to think more about the stored seeds of psychosis.

It was Greg, a successful physiotherapist, who started me off in this direction. He had always been involved in health, fitness and spirituality. Then one day he tried ecstasy, and it exploded the boundaries of his world. He wanted more. He progressed from ecstasy to speed, and then to ice. Within two years he was living for drugs. He ran up huge debts, and eventually lost his business and his home and became psychotic. He thought he was constantly being followed and would spend nights on the roof of his house or driving around in the dark trying to spot or outwit his pursuers. Greg actually enjoyed this intense, unreal and strangely addictive state.

Greg eventually got off drugs through various programs and stints in rehab centres, then developed a very disciplined life. He monitored his diet, jogged each morning and did an athletic form of yoga. He built his physiotherapy business up again and worked long but regular hours. He always had the feeling the psychosis was still there, though, so he constantly avoided situations in which he thought it might be triggered—mental overwork, excessive physical exertion, lack of rest or watching movies with mad characters or psycho themes.

The minute he said this I realised this was exactly the same in my case. There was no remarkable day when my own craziness just went away. After my grandiose delusion stage, I packed away my robes and staff, and Schroeder was relocated to a new home on a farm. I gradually progressed from being really weird to just weird, until I resembled everyone else. This process took quite a few years. But for a long time I felt as if I too had a template for 'losing it' embedded in my brain.

This is because I went through a period during which I did keep losing it. The onset of these episodes was marked by a sense of disintegration that felt like I was moving away from what was happening around me. I quickly learned to recognise the warning signs and act. Priority number one was to escape the stimuli—to get out, get back into my own space and regain a sense of centre. Better still was to avoid the situations that might set things off in the first place. These included exercising furiously, getting highly stressed, fasting or being severely hungover. Even excitement could bring it on and I had to be really careful not to get too yang about things. Sometimes I didn't have that option or left it too late, and I would shoot back up to redline weird in no time, making disconnected comments and acting abnormally.

TRANSFORMING PSYCHOSIS

It wasn't until I was explaining to Greg why he had those feelings that I understood why certain things could trigger this psychosis long after the drugs were gone. Drugs are yang. They create an excess of 'heat', which disintegrates physical form. Psychosis is an excessive heat pattern. When you are in that state everything is disordered and anarchic. Afterwards things cool down, but it is as if the heat pattern, the energy of the psychosis, gets trapped in matter like a bubble of air trapped in a block of ice. It sits there waiting to be released.

I told Greg he needed to deal with the psychosis by recreating the heat environment, so that any stored remnants could be processed and transformed.

TRAUMA RELEASE

The thing I had done that Greg hadn't was the intense spiritual training. It wasn't just the meditation. My spiritual teacher had also introduced me to a trauma release technique specifically designed to remove psychic or spiritual traumas. It begins in the same way as a normal meditation, with a sacred chant to awaken the spirit force, then you request a release of the trauma stored within. This brings the trauma to the surface, to the conscious mind. As the stored energy of the trauma meets the spirit force, the experience becomes explosive, primal and cathartic.

I would feel ecstatic, as though high voltage power was surging through every cell in my body. The motivation to move would overpower me. I would shake, roll around the floor and make strange noises. In those days it felt as if there was a heavy ball of condensed energy stuck inside and I had an uncontrollable urge to expel it, like a kind of 'spiritual vomiting'. My response to the trauma release process seemed much more powerful than for others in the group. By the end of each session I would be dripping with sweat, as if I had been running. Afterwards I felt like I had spent a month in a health spa. My whole being was light, bubbling and clear.

It wasn't until Greg sat in front of me that I realised the trauma release must have allowed me to release remnants of stored psychosis. I participated in many trauma release sessions and after each one I felt lighter. Within a year of doing this, people told me my face had changed, that the drug look was gone from my eyes. In traditional Chinese medicine, our spirit can be assessed through the eyes. In health it will be a shining light. If it is dull, withdrawn or out of control, it indicates the person has lost their spirit.[1] After a few years of doing trauma release, I never had another crazy episode.

SPIRITUAL DETOXING

The trauma release process allows the person to enter the territory of their psychosis in a safe and controlled way. This technique relies on igniting 'spiritual fire' and can be tremendously powerful. You voluntarily enter a state that, if accessed in an involuntary manner, would be called madness or psychosis. However, now you can grasp it and process it under the guidance of a higher power. You can sift out the seeds of it and release the energies.

Greg, the physiotherapist, was a suitable candidate for my spiritual detox work. He had the physical discipline to be able to balance it and the mental discipline to follow through and work with it afterwards, which is crucially important. Psychosis is an excess of energy and past drug use stores excess energy. If this has not been transformed and you add spiritual fire, it can be a 'powder keg' situation. It is easy to ignite, but requires discipline to control it afterwards.

This work is not a counselling session but a more hands-on experience. I begin by asking for guidance and protection from the highest source of good. Then I initiate the process.

When I took Greg through the process I felt the fire rising in me and waited for it to spread across to him. I could sense he was a real powder keg. Sure enough, it only took seconds for him to respond. He started panting and shaking so violently the room vibrated. Suddenly, he dropped to the floor, but instantly leapt back up again. Then he started making guttural noises that became louder and more vigorous. His voice changed, his body tensed and he started speaking gibberish.

Deep-seated unconscious material was now freely being expressed through a range of emotions, actions and sounds. As the conscious mind has no words to express such spiritual and emotional complexity, it creates its own language. When you are in that state the sounds you produce make perfect sense to you.

You are fully conscious and in control of your actions, and can stop if you want, but you don't want to because it feels so good to finally release and process the feelings. It is like the roll-up to an orgasm. It feels so right you want to see it through. All the time I am connected to the client, monitoring their progress. Through my training with my spiritual teacher, my chi-work, and decades of running group meditations, initiating and training people, I can feel exactly where the client is and can guide them.

Greg continued making the noises for a while, then started stomping on the floor, as if he was trying to break through a wall, cage or prison. This action represents 'destroying the fabric of suppression'. Then everything shifted. His actions and voice became softer and more passive. Now he was regressing, allowing himself to be a vulnerable child again. Then he switched to being assertive (yang), then changed back to passive (yin) again, reaffirming it was safe for him to be vulnerable. After about ten minutes this ceased abruptly and he seemed awestruck by something. At this stage clients have the sensation that everything is absolutely clear and makes perfect sense. With this clarity comes unimaginable joy.

Greg started laughing delightedly. Then he became quiet and totally still. By now he was soaked in sweat. The spiritual fire had done its work. I knew that the session was coming to a close. I acknowledged and requested the completion of the session by asking for the cleansing of ourselves and the room, and the removal of all heaviness and dross taken on from each other during the session. The feeling of the meditation changed instantly. An effervescent wave of energy washed through us and the room, accompanied by a beautiful lightness. I then asked to receive the gift of love and inner peace, and it was delivered. We stood there with our eyes closed soaking up the bliss for a few minutes. I uttered the closing mantra and thanked the higher power for allowing it to happen.

Greg opened his mouth but couldn't speak. He had such a stunned expression on his face that we both broke into laughter. It had only been about twenty minutes, but it was as if we had crossed the universe together. I explained that this technique had allowed him to activate and engage with the yang energies of the psychosis and the drugs. He had broken through his conditioning, expressed the suppressed parts of himself and all his emotions on the deepest possible level in the context of love and freedom. During the process there had been no one controlling him, he was totally free.

He could not believe how fantastic he felt. He sensed a significant change and knew he had something constructive to work with. I told him that with that level of healing comes responsibility. This meant he had to follow up on his goals, but also deal with everything in his life openly and honestly. This included himself, his relationships and his career.

As this process allows a conscious connection with the unconscious, it releases a lot of complex information. Over the next few weeks this information becomes clearer. I did quite a few follow-up sessions with Greg and each time his response was less dramatic. He added meditation to his daily routine of exercise, as the connection with spirit needs to be refreshed on a daily basis. It also allowed Greg to keep 'burning' residual bits of the psychosis. He said that each day he felt more clarity about his purpose and destiny. He also said he seemed to have developed powerful psychic abilities. I have seen this often in people. The drug/psychosis increases your receptivity, and the meditation can make that beneficial through transforming it into clairvoyant abilities.

For Greg, that initial spiritual detox was a much more mind-blowing experience than any drug he had taken. He opened up more about other experiences he had had, not only on ice and ecstasy, but also on ketamine, a 'dissociative anaesthetic' used in veterinary medicine. Ketamine gave him the feeling he could fly and slip into other dimensions, which he felt were spiritual or mystical states. He mentioned this in rehab but the idea was immediately dismissed as hallucinations or psychotic symptoms rather than spiritual experiences.

The debate about 'chemical versus spontaneous mysticism' is an area that most recovery programs do not examine. I think we need to bring this into future drug repair programs. In Greg's case it emerged that it was this supernatural aspect of the drugs he had really loved. He said he could 'sort of' replace what the speed or ice had provided with running and exercising intensely, but it was the altered

> The debate about 'chemical versus spontaneous mysticism' is an area that most recovery programs do not examine. I think we need to bring this into future drug repair programs.

states ketamine delivered that he craved the most. When he talked about ketamine, it was with such passion he really came alive. He imagined that by stopping drugs all of that would be gone forever from his life, but now he saw this meditation was introducing that psychedelic element back into his life.

When I talk about meditation I am not talking about sitting still and controlling the mind by imagining peaceful scenes. That is relaxation. Meditation is initiated by a master or qualified teacher and feels more like a cross between an orgasm and a speed high. The experience is so powerful you don't have to think about becoming single-minded, you are single-minded. Meditation can match and surpass any drug state. When Greg said the meditation was providing him with the type of psychedelic experiences drugs had, another piece of the post-drug high puzzle fell into place for me.

PART VIII:
POST-DRUG HIGH

36 RECAPTURING THE DREAM

As a child I wanted to be a wizard. I dreamed of having magical powers and living in a mystical landscape. Lightning would fly from my hands, otherworldly beings would swoop past me and the cosmos would spin around me. I would travel and teach people the secrets of the universe. Whenever I spoke about this dream, I was told to grow up, but once I dropped LSD, I realised I didn't have to. Drugs brought my dreams to life. Then they took them away again.

Post-drug depression brought me to my knees. I started thinking that maybe my dreams were just stupid fantasies, and I resigned myself to a half-life. Many ex-drug users do this. It is as if they concede defeat. They don't think they will ever feel as good, high or happy again. Life after drugs should not be about opting for second best. There is no limit to how good you can feel after drugs and no limit to what dreams you can achieve. You can recapture everything again without drugs. This means remembering and reviving your dreams, and once again altering your consciousness in a way that keeps increasing in intensity.

> Post-drug depression brought me to my knees. I started thinking that maybe my dreams were just stupid fantasies, and I resigned myself to a half-life. Many ex-drug users do this.

Life after drugs should not be about opting for second best. There is no limit to how good you can feel after drugs and no limit to what dreams you can achieve.

● ● ● ● ● ● ● ●

DRUGS AND SPIRITUALITY

The way to do all this is to physically live differently and follow the spiritual path. Many people turn to spirituality after a heavy recreational drug past. This will only work if you are strong and healthy, and if the spiritual experience is as intense and overwhelming as a drug experience.

Terry gave up hard drugs and tried to replace them with mass on Sundays, and it didn't work. The first time Terry walked in to my clinic I remember thinking what a 'together' person he was. He was a celebrity chef and had great charisma, great hair, great clothes and probably a nice car as well. He had that air of success—the solid, established person other people wanted to be like and drug users feel inadequate around.

Then he started talking. He had gone ten weeks without hard drugs and felt like crap. He was constantly depressed, exhausted, and either angry or on the verge of tears. He wasn't on the ball and couldn't afford to be like that. He had nothing to live for and felt like he was dead already. The only thing that excited him now was the idea of being able to feel normal again. His definition of normal was a person who is at peace, free to do what they want and able to deal with their emotions. Then I asked him who came to mind when he thought of 'normal'. He looked at me and said, 'You.' Never in my wildest dreams did I think I would be someone's ideas of 'normal'.

Terry had been prescribed antidepressants and sleeping tablets, but they made him feel weird. His doctor kept changing his prescription, but Terry believed the medication was interfering with the way he wanted to be. He wanted to feel like he did in the old days on ecstasy, speed and ice—energetic, excited, purposeful and passionate about life. His eyes lit up as he talked. From his first joint at fifteen, he was transported out of the boring suburban world and all his senses came alive. He progressed from dope to LSD, then ecstasy and speed.

When Terry reached his early twenties he was using speed on a daily basis. He loved ecstasy for the spiritual feelings it generated and would take it on weekends. He estimated he would do at least five hundred ecstasy trips a year. His life on drugs was fantastic, highly charged and exciting but then the destructive side surfaced. Terry crossed the line to needing drugs to function. This ushered in that next phase, all too familiar for most long-term hard-drug users, when you start battling the negative energy of drugs. His wife, who also worked in hospitality, was equally passionate about drugs, but her passion had led to heroin addiction.

CONVENTIONAL SPIRITUALITY

By the time he was twenty-five, Terry realised that he and his wife were on an express train to destruction. The drugs were draining their money and eroding their health, integrity and relationship. They urgently needed a major change. Terry had been raised in a religious household, so he decided he would draw on his faith to pull them out of the abyss.

He and his wife gave up drugs and started going to church. Terry tried to pray and live a good life, but he didn't think he could live up to the church people or the teachings of the church. Every time he went to mass or associated with other members of the congregation he felt guilty, contaminated, and a sinner. That environment was a constant reminder of what he wasn't. During that time his marriage broke up, he put on twenty kilos, was totally stressed-out and drained, and only had enough energy to go to work. No matter how much he prayed or how many times he went to mass, he couldn't feel the sense of support and belonging that drugs had provided.

After a few years Terry left the church and started using drugs again. Within months he was using speed on a daily basis, and ice as well. He did feel terrific for a while, as if his real self had come back, until the side-effects returned, at which point he dropped back to weekend drug use. By then his weekdays were a living nightmare. He was scattered, depressed, anxious and fearful. The fear was the worst part. Every booking evoked fear. Every function he had to cater created fear. He could barely face going to work each day because of the fear. He only made it through the week because he knew he could take drugs on the weekend and get some relief. The weekend was his ticket out of hell. After a while he couldn't handle the side-effects anymore and had to give up the weekend drug use as well. In the ten weeks since then, he had been stuck in hell.

A NEW APPROACH

I asked how he spent a typical day from when he woke up to when he went to bed. He was currently on day shifts. He got up at 7 am feeling tired, anxious and fearful that the day would get out of control. He had to be at work by 7:45 am. Between waking up and getting in the car he had about twenty minutes. Anxiety prevented him from being able to eat so, after a quick shower, he gulped down several cups of coffee and had three or four cigarettes, then he rushed to work to try and get things under control.

Throughout the day he felt tired, as if he had no support. He had no appetite. It took him ages to swallow food so he would nibble on greasy, salty or sweet snacks rather than eat proper meals. In the afternoons, he would have a few energy soft drinks. By the time he got home he was aggravated and annoyed. He would also be exhausted, but unable to sleep unless he was medicated.

> Drugs show us the solution is within us. Instead of trying to control the external world, Terry needed to focus on controlling his internal world. He had to do naturally what drugs do artificially—create chi flow and enhance his organ function.

Most of Terry's side-effects were due to organ depletion and his current lifestyle was exacerbating the problem. As he felt out of control, he became a control freak with his staff. He knew if he had a line of cocaine at work everything would change in a second. He would feel in charge and things would flow smoothly. But the only thing that would have changed after snorting cocaine was Terry's internal world. Drugs show us the solution is within us. Instead of trying to control the external world, Terry needed to focus on controlling his internal world. He had to do naturally what drugs do artificially—create chi flow and enhance his organ function.

I devised a diet, exercise and therapy program for him which he followed to the letter. Within weeks there were marked improvements in his physical and emotional health, so in the following therapy sessions we moved on to the spiritual aspect as it was obvious Terry didn't really want to just feel normal, he wanted to feel extraordinary again, the way the early drug experiences had made him feel before the hard drugs turned it all bad. He didn't know it was possible to feel extraordinary again.

As they had for Terry, drugs had shown me magic and my place in the cosmos. I felt connected, complete and satisfied. That resonated so deeply with my soul I wanted more and more of it. The psychedelics couldn't keep delivering though, so I turned to speed and it was the beginning of the end. Desperation, addiction and despair broke me, and afterwards I too longed just to be normal. But after a drug history like mine, or Terry's, you have to aim your sights a whole lot higher than normal; you have to want to be extraordinary again, and this is possible.

It was obvious Terry didn't really want to just feel normal, he wanted to feel extraordinary again, the way the early drug experiences had made him feel before the hard drugs turned it all bad. He didn't know it was possible to feel extraordinary again.

After a drug history like mine, or Terry's, you have to aim your sights a whole lot higher than normal; you have to want to be extraordinary again, and this is possible.

37 OTHER DIMENSIONS

Terry loved drugs because they made him feel connected and supported. When he gave up he hoped church would replace these feelings, but it didn't. It didn't provide him with an alternative to drugs, because most churches have become bland. Terry was left feeling separation and loss. His post-drug pain and fear were unbearable. He wanted that pain to go away, and needed to build his inner energy and improve his organ health to get his symptoms under control, but what he also needed was that sense of ecstasy and union again.

So, his soul-satisfaction had to be found in alternative models of spirituality. Spiritual practice is much more powerful than drugs. In my daily practice I now feel the same dream-like quality of being asleep while awake that I loved about marijuana, and I can experience states that are like a mix of cocaine and LSD all at once. Everything I had wanted was there all along and I didn't have to take a drug to get it. I can go there at will. Each meditation takes me to a wonderful world and each time it is different, just like drug trips. So, each day now has the

> Each meditation takes me to a wonderful world and each time it is different, just like drug trips. So, each day now has the potential to deliver an even more beautiful and profound experience than the last.

potential to deliver an even more beautiful and profound experience than the last.

THE MEDITATION WORLD

As soon as I finish invoking the meditation I am instantly transported to a mystical landscape. In the deep blue twilight, a silver lake ringed by huge mountains lies before me and stars circle around me. Beings gather and fire energy into my heart. It charges through my cells and shoots out of my fingertips. I am disintegrating but reintegrating at the same time. I feel overwhelming love.

Now everything is becoming light around me. I am in a different place, maybe another dimension. It is a glowing golden yellow. This place is warm, comforting and nourishing, and infinite. I can be anywhere in an instant, just by thinking of it. I am told this is my home. This is who I am. A very sacred feeling washes over me and I am in a state of prayer. I immerse myself in it and surrender to it. I know the nature of the cosmos is pure love. If we knew how much love there was we would never have another dark thought.

OTHER DIMENSIONS

These are not hallucinations or archetypes from my subconscious, and my ability to access these places is not drug induced. These realms exist and are more real than material reality. My childhood dreams of wondrous worlds in other dimensions were, in fact, realistic. This sounds very trippy but even scientists are now taking a wider view of reality. In some fields of physics it is being proposed that the structure of our universe is not simply three-dimensional. Superstring theories postulate that there are many other dimensions of time and space existing

These are not hallucinations or archetypes from my subconscious, and my ability to access these places is not drug induced. These realms exist and are more real than material reality. My childhood dreams of wondrous worlds in other dimensions were, in fact, realistic.

in the universe. Recent research in physics that extends string theory has led to the development of the M-theory, or membrane theory, and draws on the idea of parallel universes and multiple dimensions.[1] The renowned physicist Edward Witten, who developed the M-theory, suggests our universe could be sitting on a membrane in some higher dimensional space.[2]

A multi-dimensional universe is hardly a new discovery. In cultures in which people practice methods of chi cultivation and seek enlightenment, the existence of other dimensions was accepted thousands of years ago. While some dismiss these possibilities, a much larger portion of the population, many of whom have had drug experiences, have also experienced other realms and dimensions. For some full recovery means reclaiming that knowledge and going back to those worlds. This means making spiritual practices a key part of life after drugs.

DRUGS AND THE REAL WORLD

Andrew had been using drugs since he was seventeen. He had been an excellent student but school didn't engage him, so he dropped out. Then he discovered drugs and a world that excited him. He loved magic mushrooms, LSD, ecstasy and speed, because they could take him to other places and make him feel 'right'.

When they stopped doing this he quit. Then life was so empty he took up speed again. Andrew started living for speed. He would work drug-free for three weeks on oil rigs, followed by a few ecstatic days high on speed. After sleeping for one night he would go back to work. Then he'd count off the days until he could take drugs again. He only did the job so he could afford the speed to escape the dull world he was trapped in.

Andrew finally quit, but without speed he felt confused, depressed and couldn't sleep, so he was put on medication. Everyone around him had houses, mortgages and families and part of him felt he had thrown his life away and that it was too late to get it back. At the same time he didn't want to be a professional with a house in the suburbs. Drugs had shown him a much better reality, but that world went with the drugs so he felt his only option was to go back to the normal world he hated.

I explained to Andrew that according to the spiritual masters the material world most people live in is the false world and the real world is the world of spirit. We have the choice to operate within the boundaries of the false world, or to make the leap into the real world.

Andrew's depression, insomnia and restlessness were due to organ destruction from excessive speed use, but they were also a result of him feeling trapped and lost. He was in no man's land, just as I had been. So I explained that when I took drugs I too believed the magical place they took me to was the real world, but at the same time I knew the experience was somehow false, because it was drug-induced. It was as if I had been watching a fantastic movie but then had to walk out of the cinema and back into bland suburban reality.

BORING, BORING, BORING

After drugs I had a long struggle with these different realities and kept trying to fit back into the normal/false world. But I couldn't. Initially I thought it was because I was depressed, depleted or screwed-up, but even after I was no longer quite as depressed and screwed-up, I still felt the same. The truth was, after all my time in the drug world, the normal world was excruciatingly boring.

Parents always tell me that they can't understand why their children need drugs. They ask why they can't enjoy nature or go for a run to feel high. But once you have done drugs and seen nature being created in an explosion of technicoloured mind-blowing glory, bushwalking is not going to do it for you, particularly if you are depleted, as your world view automatically defaults to negative.

I always thought there was something wrong with me for not being able to enjoy the normal world after drugs, for thinking it was boring. Then one of my lecturers told me about a talk he had attended by a renowned tai-chi master. After the talk someone asked the master what the purpose of tai-chi was, and apparently he answered 'to alleviate boredom'. The audience looked surprised but his response makes sense for ex-drug users. We are living in a world of extraordinary technological progress and this has improved our lives immeasurably, but we don't have any interactions with the world of spirit.

After drugs we need techniques to open the doors to those worlds again, to put some magic back into life. My salvation came from discovering that I could go back there, it just took me a very long time to understand that to do this I had to walk through the door. This was what Andrew was going to have to do, along with all the other accelerated, intense, visionary young people like him. I asked Andrew what he would have thought of a school where they taught the levitating skills of the yogis, then used physics and biology to interpret it. His eyes lit up. He said he would have loved that. He had read the *Autobiography of a Yogi* and was fascinated by ancient mysticism. But those schools don't exist. As a child you can't learn about the magic of your organs, other dimensions and the expansion of the spirit. If you could, drug consumption would drop dramatically.

As a child you can't learn about the magic of your organs, other dimensions and the expansion of the spirit. If you could, drug consumption would drop dramatically.

● ● ● ● ● ● ● ●

38 A DOORWAY TO THE FUTURE

New recreational drugs will continue to be developed to try and reach new frontiers of euphoria and bliss, but no matter how sophisticated the technology, there will always be savage side-effects. The simple truth is that these substances will never reach the power and intensity of what the human body and the creative forces of the universe can deliver.

If people understood what they could achieve with their own body they would lose interest in drugs. Spiritual teachings tell us that most of us are oblivious to our true nature and potential. Our spirit has no limitations. This is how we are designed to function. But life throws up constant challenges for us and we face ongoing shock, pain and trauma. Our inability to deal with these things creates blockages in our energy field. For many of us this begins in early childhood as our dreams and our spiritual nature are suppressed. By the time we are adults, our organs no longer have the abundant flow of chi that we had as young children. Instead they are depleted and cannot provide the bliss, love, euphoria and ability to live in the present that is our birthright. Recreational drugs flush the system with so much life energy or chi that

> If people understood what they could achieve with their own body they would lose interest in drugs.

it rushes past the blockages and floods the organs. This instantly reminds us of our true nature. The veil is temporarily lifted but the cost is high.

THE STONED APES

Some researchers propose that hallucinogenic drugs created a leap in human evolution. Terence McKenna's 'stoned ape' theory suggests that the quick tripling of brain size that occurred among some primates 1.5 million years ago, and that made us self-aware humans, occurred as a result of primate psyche-delic drug experiences. As our tree-dwelling primate ancestors took up a life out in the open, hallucinogenic mushrooms became part of their diet. This modified their behaviour and led to self-awareness, which in turn led to the development of spoken language and imagination.[1] When subsequent climate changes removed the mushroom from the human diet, McKenna believes we reverted to pre-mushroom brutal primate social structures.[2]

Behaviour-modifying drugs are back in our diet in a significant manner. They have 'reappeared' in a modern, rational and scientific culture at a time when we have become separated from the natural world and dismissive of magic and mysticism. Perhaps, despite the pain and destruction linked with drug use, we now have an opportunity to make good of it. If we continue the journey of spiritual discovery in life after drugs we can create another positive evolutionary shift in consciousness.

DRUGS AS AN EVOLUTIONARY TOOL

I am firmly convinced that drugs can be an evolutionary tool. High on drugs, you can feel self-realised. You see what your organs are capable of delivering. If in post-drug life you stick to the plan of 'beginning with the end in mind' and seek to recapture those states without drugs, you will evolve.

A question I often put to my clients is—if monkeys plus mushrooms equals man, what does man plus mushrooms equal? If it was psychedelic substances that led to self-awareness and the development of language and ultimately our communications-based society, what could be salvaged from the devastation of the drug epidemic? The monkeys ate the mushrooms and became self-aware—could we convert drug pasts into a catalyst for self-realisation? Once the monkey eats the mushrooms and gains self-awareness, it can't turn back. This is the same for people who have had revelatory drug experiences. You can't change the past and there is no point trying to go back to where you were before. You need to go fearlessly forward.

THE DEATH OF THE PSYCHE

Of course this does leave open the question that if drugs are an evolutionary tool, why not just take drugs and evolve? Unfortunately this is not how it works. What I have learned is that the old has to go before the new can develop. This must be done *consciously* within your body and within your lifetime. This means you may have to go through painful physical, emotional and spiritual experiences. You have to be prepared to have everything stripped away, to get to your innermost core of pain to allow your deepest wounds to heal.

> You can't change the past and there is no point trying to go back to where you were before. You need to go fearlessly forward.

My post-drug high came at the cost of what I now see as a series of psychic deaths. I underwent a long process of shedding layers of pain, like skins. The release of each layer was marked by physical and spiritual symptoms. I still experience this process but understand it as part of the journey. I know that once I allow the healing to happen, the reward will be access to a new level of awareness and inner peace.

The last incident occurred when I was so physically weak I had to spend a few days in bed. This is a rare occurrence for me and I think it happened for a reason. I ended up going back into some unresolved emotional territory. I was hearing voices and seeing things, weird stuff, not nice stuff. I felt as if I was losing my mind.

It wasn't until the morning of the fifth day that I could feel a lifting of the dread. I slowly got up to do some meditation. I was so weak and dizzy that each step was hard work. I placed my hands on my knees, palms upwards. Within seconds of beginning the meditation, the most sacred feeling I had ever had swept through me. I could feel a feather-light touch on my fingers. Two beings in front of me took my hands and poured life force into them. This stabilised me and gave me the strength to go into a deeper meditation. I stood up and surrendered myself to it. All the weakness disappeared. After about ten minutes I sensed another presence. A much larger being, about two and a half metres high, appeared in front of me and engulfed me in a deep, deep healing. Overwhelming feelings of love coursed through me. In that moment I realised that this was my first conscious experience with an angel.

I fell to my knees in awe. I hate to say it, but it was very similar to the experience I'd had many years earlier when I received my mission with my goat, Schroeder, and swore to follow the path of good. But this time it was from a place of mind, body and spirit integration, and was so real it vibrated through my every cell.

Then the soul pain erupted from the core of my being. I had buried it so deeply I had never been able to reach it before. But the five days of illness had emptied everything from my body and it finally surfaced. The memories of my mother and her suffering hit me first. I could see the agony in her eyes that day she thought I was going to die, and how I sneered at her pain and embraced the darkness. I broke down and cried more deeply than I ever had. I felt heart-stabbing convulsive grief over my best friend's death in Germany, my culpability for abandoning him, and the agony of the thought of him dying sad and alone. Then images roiled up from my subconscious and flashed before my eyes: the junkies in the squats in Amsterdam, the sickening reptiles, the eyes of a young guy whose face was being razor-slashed by drug dealers, the terrible day I decided to die. As each image rose up before me I affirmed that I was a soul of the light.

Then the pain of the drug users I treat, and that of their parents and friends and family, surfaced. I finally understood the infinite universe of pain that comes with drug use. Each story I hear from a patient is one of heartbreak, loss and alienation from their true nature, and all the terrible destruction and devastation of the drug world tore out of me in great shattering sobs from the depths of my being until finally there was nothing left. I was empty. I felt healed, physically, spiritually and emotionally, as if I had undergone a transformation and had at last redeemed my soul.

THE BEGINNING

I thought I had resolved my past simply by admitting to it and writing *Higher and Higher*. To some extent I had, but there was so much more. If you do hard drugs the way I did, it closes off your heart. This creates deep inner pain. We devote so much time and effort to avoiding pain, we don't understand its composition. My subsequent years spent talking and thinking almost exclusively about drugs and pain enabled me to see that my pain was not only the physical, spiritual and emotional pain of depleted organs, but also the bad memories of walking on the dark side. I also think many drug users can open up to the collective consciousness of pain.

In a recent meditation I asked for guidance about what had happened to me over those five days. The image that appeared was a massive locked vault door and a key to open it. I thought I had faced my deep-seated pain in my 'walking the black dog' days, but I now understood there were layers of the stuff. I had worked on the outer layers, but the five days of processing allowed access to the core of my pain, so I could acknowledge it and resolve it. This was done by unconditionally accepting the worst parts of myself. Once you do that the pain doesn't hurt anymore.

FEAR AND LOATHING AND SELF-LOVE

Back when I went through the trauma release process with my spiritual teacher, I felt I was purging something from myself. However, I didn't understand the transformational potential of drugs then. I was still caught up in the idea that I had done something bad and had to cleanse myself. I'd missed the point. I see now I was not supposed to get rid of some part of me I didn't want anymore, it was supposed to be about transforming, accepting and integrating that into myself.

I had never confronted my really bad memories and they had to surface one way or another. I had to accept all of that as a part of me, an extension of myself. Ultimately it was about self-acceptance. Self-acceptance is connected with self-worth and self-worth is connected to self-love. It always seemed such a fluffy concept, but now I believe accepting or loving yourself comes by doing things that build self-worth. This means doing things you fear, so it is by facing your fear that you turn your pain into love.

> Self-acceptance is connected with self-worth and self-worth is connected to self-love. It always seemed such a fluffy concept, but now I believe accepting or loving yourself comes by doing things that build self-worth. This means doing things you fear, so it is by facing your fear that you turn your pain into love.

● ● ● ● ● ● ● ●

My greatest fear was public speaking. It was a pathological fear based on actual post-drug experiences of blanking out in front of groups of people. As a student in my first semester of college, when I was still battling chronic fear on a daily basis, I made sure I never drew attention to myself. One day I got sick of that and boldly put up my hand to ask a question. The teacher asked me what my question was. Everyone turned around to look at me and suddenly I was in a vacuum, I couldn't speak. There was no air, I couldn't breathe. I had to run out of the room.

As I took more Chinese herbs and built up my organs, over time I became capable of physically overcoming the fear, but those memories never left me. On my first promotional tour, my fear was so intense that I nearly backed out. People said 'you'll be fine', but drug users' fears are real, because they have to combat real memories of things not being fine. I knew the only way forward was to create real scenarios where new memories could be born, so I made myself do talks, workshops, live-to-air radio interviews and debates. I spoke in shopping centers, at festivals and conferences, whether there was one person in the audience or hundreds. Each time I had to overcome a solid wall of sickening fear, but each time a little more self-worth and self-acceptance crept in. As my excitement and inspiration increased, my ingrained image of myself as scum finally lost some of its power, and a side of myself I liked slowly came forward.

Facing and overcoming my fears was an essential part of my journey. As I kept facing more fear, things kept moving. The energy built and built. As I became more at ease with the idea of pain and spoke more openly in public about how crazy I had been, I attracted clients who had also accelerated the onset of such pain. The only option was to go into it and evolve. In the counselling sessions I took them into the centre of their pain, which in turn brought me closer to the core of my own pain. If I hadn't overcome the fear I wouldn't have processed my soul pain. Everything was worth it for that.

39 THE POST-DRUG HIGH PROGRAM

For all drug users who no longer want drugs but still want something more than the normal world, the solution is to embark on the spiritual path. The way you begin to do this is through the physical, by rebuilding the organs. As you slowly change your body you become sensitised to subtle energy fields and communications, and guidance from the spiritual realms.

I work with a customised practice that builds strength while laying the foundation for accessing altered states. My program blends chi-cultivating techniques, meditation, endurance and weight training with success strategies. I draw from many traditions, but apply their teachings in non-traditional ways.

Often clients follow a program I provide and take up martial arts but the instructors will tell them not to do the weight training I recommended as it interferes with their martial art performance. This is because martial arts utilise tendons, whereas weight training emphasises muscles, and building muscle can affect martial art fighting skills. Likewise with yoga, there are certain schools that do not recommend endurance training because that element is already encompassed in the yoga form. But, as I explain to my clients, we are not doing these practices to become a master of martial arts or a yogi or guru in the traditional manner. We are seeking to be what I call a post-drug master. It is a *new* path.

BEGINNING WITH THE END IN MIND

Drug users are a different kind of spiritual student on many levels. Firstly many have had a preview of the end goal. We have had out-of-body experiences, visions and states of bliss and profound fulfilment. The upside of amazing drug-induced experiences—of being euphoric, loving, abundant and feeling expansion in accord with the universe—is that you can begin the spiritual path with the end in mind. However, because you know what's coming, you also need it faster than other people. You need the spiritual equivalent of intravenous delivery and accelerated results.

This acceleration comes through a mixture of practices and techniques. I have seen a lot of former drug-using clients become spiritual junkies, addicted to the bliss and euphoria of meditative states, but who neglect their bodies. Many end up so 'out there' they might as well be using speed. The post-drug path to spirituality has to be based on the step-by-step repetition inherent in the traditional chi-cultivating forms. If you go directly to the state transmitted by a spiritual master as if it was a drug high with no physical groundwork, it can create confusion and leave you feeling fragmented. To be a post-drug master, you have to train in the basics every day, and refresh the end goal every day with meditation.

> I have seen a lot of former drug-using clients become spiritual junkies, addicted to the bliss and euphoria of meditative states, but who neglect their bodies. Many end up so 'out there' they might as well be using speed.

THE PHYSICAL/SPIRITUAL MATCH

I never recommend any practice or product unless I have tested it on myself. It took me a long time to develop this customised approach, but as I followed my intuition and allowed myself to make changes to traditional forms, the beneficial effects on my health were immediately evident. I have spent as much time now on the spiritual path as I did on the drug path, and I have to say I have more consistent and incredible highs with this practice than I ever had on drugs, but only because I keep the physical basics going.

What I finally understood was that you have to balance the heightened awareness and visions (yang) with the physical (yin). I can only work with my increased receptivity because I have matched it with increased physical engagement. The further out you go in your mind, the more intense the involvement of your body needs to be. Yogis practise extreme physical control to match their extreme spiritual activity.

> The further out you go in your mind, the more intense the involvement of your body needs to be. Yogis practise extreme physical control to match their extreme spiritual activity.

MEDITATION

Doing my practice every day generates altered states far beyond anything I could have imagined on drugs. When I invoke the meditative state each morning an uplifting feeling washes over me, mixed with the disintegration of form that many of my psychedelic drug trips began with. I hear sounds like bells chiming and my body feels weightless. It is like the high of LSD, which is an incredibly pleasurable feeling. Everything around me in the material world becomes transparent. Objects appear holographic—I am sure I could pass my hand right through them. My body feels as if I was just one step away from levitation and could float up to the sky.

In a traditional spiritual practice this experience would end after about thirty minutes. But I want to bring it into my body, otherwise it is purely in my head. So I align the spiritual experience with my body by holding the altered state while doing a kind of martial tai-chi. I alternate between attacking (yang) and gathering (yin), so the spiritual clarity from the meditation is put into the physical context of action. Now I feel invincible, charged up, but calm as well, like I'm on good speed. I also feel grounded but ready to move in an instant and engage with anything.

I also integrate the spiritual into the physical by continuing to maintain the state derived from the meditation and tai-chi while running. This engages my lungs more intensively and puts me completely into the now. Then I add the weights work. I sink deeply into my muscles and convert body/mind resistance into acceptance. This brings the whole practice to a peak and I experience myself as pure power, pure will and in the present. Everything I ever got from any drug I feel right now. I know who I am, I know my purpose and the universe is open to me. This is a high that never stops.

> Everything I ever got from any drug I feel right now. I know who I am, I know my purpose and the universe is open to me. This is a high that never stops.

POST-DRUG HIGH

Throughout the day I constantly monitor and work with my inner energy. If I have an important meeting in the morning, whether professional or personal, while commut-

ing I hold the state generated by my practice and draw upon strong kidney energies for willpower to combat fear, and healthy spleen energies for focus and fluid consistency of speech and thoughts. In the meeting I can call upon a bright burning fire element in order to experience joy and love, independent of the external situation. This gives me confidence, as I am not attached to outcomes.

By lunchtime I want to get the best out of the food I eat, so I call upon metal energies to cut through all stressful thoughts. This enables me to live in the now and have an empty mind so I can concentrate on the food and on enjoying it. This delivers a maximum supply of nutrients, so I feel recharged and at inner peace.

There is not a moment in the day when I am not aware of the existence of other dimensions. I feel a presence with me at all times, which becomes much more noticeable when I do public speaking or work with clients. In these interactions I feel spirit moving through me, so my work is also a blissful experience. I am constantly surrounded by beings that seem like old friends but not ones from any physical dimension. If I need direction with a work, life or family issue I ask for guidance.

At other times I can feel the presence of my parents, who both died some time ago. We communicate non-verbally. They are not separated from me. None of us is separated from each other. I don't ever feel alone anymore. I see now that I never was, but I was so attached to the material world that I had no idea I was connected to everyone and everything. If I want a purely psychedelic experience I can sit in a park, draw upon my ability to alter my state naturally, and suddenly even the dullest environment will vibrate in pulsating glorious colours.

> I don't ever feel alone anymore. I see now that I never was, but I was so attached to the material world that I had no idea I was connected to everyone and everything. If I want a purely psychedelic experience I can sit in a park, draw upon my ability to alter my state naturally, and suddenly even the dullest environment will vibrate in pulsating glorious colours.

CREATIVITY

Another crucial component of the post-drug high is creativity. I set aside an hour a day to work on electronic music. When I compose, I feel the presence around me very strongly. Sometimes it is an audience sitting with me and at other times it is more active. I have experienced instances in which slider positions change or the recording is altered, which always improves what I am doing, without my direct input. At other times I have the sensation that I am playing my keyboard in an almost trance-like state, and I feel my hands are guided automatically across the keys. –

Creativity resonates with the heart and has tremendous healing power. In *Hands of Light*, Barbara Ann Brennan discusses an ex-drug user client of hers who had undergone such profound self-development that he had achieved the goals he had set for his lifetime and was able to reincarnate into the same body without having to go through death and rebirth. In a conversation with her spiritual guide the message to this client was that after we finish the round of incarnations on the physical plane, healing on higher levels becomes creativity. Transformation no longer focuses on pain, but will encompass movement, music and art.[1]

NIGHT MEDITATION

I carry my altered state right through until evening. In the old days I would lie in bed at night and smoke hashish. The drug would move through me creating a sensation of simultaneously floating and sinking. I would fall towards sleep on waves of bliss. Now I end each day with a night meditation that creates effects just like the hash used to, but, unlike the hash, it keeps increasing in intensity. It generates sleep so deep that often the next thing I know I am waking up just before the alarm goes off in the morning. Then the whole process starts all over again. I now live in the world of magic. This was what I always wanted. As long as I keep my daily practice going it will never stop. There is a limit to how high you can get on drugs, but no limit to how high you can get afterwards.

Drugs are there for a reason: nothing is random. Back when I started taking drugs everyone used to talk about 'opening the doors' but I never knew what that really meant. I now think drugs open the doors to other dimensions, to spirituality and to achieving your dreams. But you can only make the experience valuable if you walk through the doors you have opened. This means going through the fear, facing the pain and accepting all parts of yourself, then going after your dream. And you can only do that if you build your body.

> I now live in the world of magic. This was what I always wanted. As long as I keep my daily practice going it will never stop. There is a limit to how high you can get on drugs, but no limit to how high you can get afterwards.

Healthy organs are the starting point to recapture the altered states, the inter-dimensional travel and the ability to expand and create in accord with our spiritual destiny. If all the hundreds of millions of current and ex-drug users committed themselves to rebuilding their body and following the path of self-realisation, not only would they recapture everything drugs have shown them, but they would change the future of the planet as well.

ENDNOTES

INTRODUCTION

1 R Davenport-Hines, 2002, *The Pursuit of Oblivion: A Social History of Drugs*, Phoenix Press, London.

2 M Males, 2007, 'This is your brain on drugs, Dad', *New York Times*, 3 January, http://www.nytimes.com/2007/01/03/opinion/03males.html.

3 T Dalrymple, 2006, *Romancing Opiates: Pharmacological Lies and the Addiction Bureaucracy*, Encounter Books, New York, p. 2.

4 A Letcher, 2006, *Shroom: A Cultural History of the Magic Mushroom*, Faber and Faber, London.

5 J Holland, 2001, *Ecstasy: The Complete Guide*, Park Street Press, Rochester, Vermont, p. 18.

6 The United Nations Office on Drugs and Crime, 2004, 'UNODC World Drug Report 2004', United Nations, Vienna.

7 L Iverson, 2006, *Speed, Ecstasy, Ritalin: The Science of Amphetamines*, Oxford University Press, Oxford.

CHAPTER 2

1 R Sheldrake, 1988, *The Presence of the Past*, Times Books, New York.

2 R Sheldrake, 1994, *The Rebirth of Nature: The Greening of Science and God*, Park Street Press, Rochester, Vermont.

3 Holland, op. cit.

CHAPTER 3

1 E Laszlo, T Pfeiffer and J Mack (eds), 2007, 'Elements of the new concept of consciousness', in *Mind Before Matter: Visions of a New Science of Consciousness*, O Books, Winchester, p. 85.

2 M Chia and T Huang, 2002, *The Secret Teachings of the Tao Te Ching*, Destiny Books, Vermont, p. 59.

3 L Hammer, 1990, *Dragon Rises Red Bird Flies: Psychology and Chinese Medicine*, Station Hill Press, New York, p. 6.

4 R Tiqua, 1996, *Traditional Chinese Medicine: A Guide to its Practice*, Choice Books, Marrickville, New South Wales, p. 35.

5 M Sankey, 1999, *Esoteric Acupuncture: Gateway to Expanded Healing*, Vol 1, Mountain Castle Publishing, California.

6 Chia and Huang, op. cit., pp. 59–60.

CHAPTER 4

1 Hammer, op. cit., p. 9.

CHAPTER 5

1 S Grof, 2006, *When the Impossible Happens: Adventures in Non-ordinary Realities*, Sounds True, Boulder, Colorado, p. 224.

2 S Gaskin, 1980, *Amazing Dope Tales*, Ronin, Berkeley, California, p. 125.

CHAPTER 10

1 G Maciocia, 1989, *The Foundations of Chinese Medicine*, Churchill Livingstone, New York, p. 80.

CHAPTER 13

1 A Shulgin and A Shulgin, 1991, *Phikal: A Chemical Love Story*, Transform Press, Berkeley, California, p. 237.

CHAPTER 20

1 B Brennan, 1988, *Hands of Light: A Guide to Healing Through the Human Energy Field*, Bantam Books, New York.

CHAPTER 22

1   Y Paramahansa, 1950, *Autobiography of a Yogi*, Rider, London.
2   Maciocia, op. cit.
3   A Escohotado, 1996, *A Brief History of Drugs: From the Stone Age to the Stoned Age*, Park Street Press, Rochester, Vermont, p. 7.

CHAPTER 23

1   T McKenna, 1993, *True Hallucinations and the Archaic Revival*, MJF, New York, p. 45.
2   R Evans Schultes and A Hofmann, 1992, *Plants of the Gods: Their Sacred, Healing and Hallucinogenic Powers*, Healing Arts Press, Rochester, Vermont, p. 148.
3   P Lamborn Wilson, 1999, *Ploughing the Clouds: The Search for Irish Soma*, City Lights, San Francisco.
4   R Winslow, 2006, 'Go ask Alice: mushroom drug is studied anew', *Wall Street Journal* online, 11 June, http://online.wsj.com/article/SB11525828044869 02994.html.

CHAPTER 24

1   Brennan, op. cit., p. 24.

CHAPTER 27

1   D Smith, 2007, *Muses, Madmen and Prophets: Rethinking the History, Science and Meaning of Auditory Hallucinations*, Penguin, New York, p. 10.

CHAPTER 28

1   Iverson, op. cit.
2   PH Connell, 1958, *Amphetamine Psychosis*, Chapman and Hall, London.
3   J Healey (ed.), 2007, 'Amphetamine use', *Issues in Society*, Vol 259, Spinney Press, New South Wales, p. 27.

CHAPTER 31

1   R Strassman, 2001, *DMT: The Spirit Molecule*, Park Street Press, Rochester, Vermont, p. 313.

CHAPTER 32

1   S Plant, 1999, *Writing on Drugs*, Farrar, Straus and Giroux, New York.
2   M Small, 2006, *The Culture of Our Discontent: Beyond the Medical Model of Mental Illness*, Joseph Henry Press, Washington DC, p. 44.

CHAPTER 33

1   Smith, op. cit., p. 130.
2   LH Diller, 2006, *The Last Normal Child: Essays on the Intersection of Kids, Culture and Psychiatric Drugs*, Praeger, Westport, Connecticut, pp. 9–10.

CHAPTER 34

1   S Grof, 2000, *The Psychology of the Future*, State University of New York Press, Albany, New York, p. 137.

CHAPTER 35

1   Hammer, op. cit.

CHAPTER 37

1   M Duffy, 1998, 'The theory formerly known as strings', *Scientific American*, February, pp. 64–9, http://www.nikhef.nl/pub/services/biblio/bib_KR/sciam14395569.pdf.
2   A Jha, 2005, 'String fellows', *Guardian*, 20 January, http://www.guardian.co.uk/science/2005/jan/20/science.research.

CHAPTER 38

1   T McKenna, 1992, *Food of the Gods*, Rider, London.
2   'Terence McKenna's "stoned ape" theory of human evolution', http//users.lycaeum.org/~sputnik/McKenna/Evolution.

CHAPTER 39

1   Brennan, op. cit., pp. 261–3.

ACKNOWLEDGEMENTS

Foremost to my wife Kirsten, without whom this book would not exist.

Maggie Hamilton, at Allen & Unwin, for believing in my vision and for her ongoing support as well as her commitment and passion to make the world a better place.

My father-in-law, Bryon Fitzpatrick, for providing support, stodge and storage space in the garage.

Karina Averlon Thomas, for enthusiastically spreading the message and contributing in so many ways.

Elizabeth Stephens, editor of *Living Now*, for publishing a series of articles outlining my controversial ideas about recreational drug repair.

Saul Fitzpatrick for the great feedback on the first draft.

To all my clients for giving me an opportunity to learn and grow.